THE
HEART & SOUL
OF SEX

THE HEART & SOUL OF SEX

Exploring the Sexual Mysteries

GINA OGDEN, PH.D.

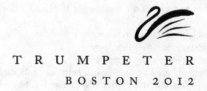

TRUMPETER
BOSTON 2012

This book is intended as an educational volume only, not as a medical manual. The information given here is designed to help you make informed decisions about your health and pleasure. It is not intended as a substitute for any treatment that may have been prescribed by your doctor. If you experience emotional discomfort or suspect that you have a medical problem, we urge you to seek competent medical help, or counseling from a skilled sexuality educator or therapist.

Trumpeter Books
An imprint of Shambhala Publications, Inc.
Horticultural Hall
300 Massachusetts Avenue
Boston, Massachusetts 02115
trumpeterbooks.com

9 8 7 6 5 4 3 2 1

First Paperback Edition
Printed in the United States of America

⊗ This edition is printed on acid-free paper that meets the
American National Standards Institute z39.48 Standard.
♻ Shambhala Publications makes every effort to print on recycled paper.
For more information please visit www.shambhala.com.
Distributed in the United States by Random House, Inc.,
and in Canada by Random House of Canada Ltd

A portion of the author's proceeds will be donated to organizations
promoting women's health.

Designed by Dede Cummings Designs

The Library of Congress catalogues the hardcover edition of this book as follows:

Ogden, Gina
The heart and soul of sex: making the ISIS connection/Gina Ogden.—1st ed.
p. cm.
Includes bibliographical references.
ISBN 978-1-59030-294-1 (hardcover)
ISBN 978-1-59030-456-3 (paperback)
1. Women—United States—Sexual behavior. 2. Sexual behavior
surveys—United States. 3. Sex (Psychology) 4. Sex—Religious aspects.
I. Title.
HQ29.O3782006
306.7082—dc22
2006000189

To all the respondents of the ISIS survey—

may your words move mountains

CONTENTS

PART TWO:

PATHS TO THE HEART AND SOUL OF SEX

INTRODUCTION
Listening to Women

As a sex therapist and researcher, I've had the privilege of listening to thousands of women describe the most intimate aspects of their lives. The more I listen the more I understand that sexual experience encompasses much more than what happens in the bedroom. It can affect our whole existence—and can become a powerful path to growth and healing.

Sex is more than something we do. Sexual energy is part of who we are, though we may not always be aware of it. Many women speak of sex as a kind of ongoing journey that changes how they respond to the world around them. Their stories range from ecstatic confluences of body, heart, and soul to chronicles of hurt, disappointment, and abuse. And many women also speak of holding back, so they experience only a tiny fraction of their sexual desire and potential.

Whatever our experiences of sex, and whatever our age, cultural background, or sexual orientation, it's almost impossible for any of us to tell the whole story. We simply don't have the language to convey the full range of our sexual feelings, our longings, fears, or dreams of what might be. Our fast-lane culture sexualizes everything from beer to Barbie, but it doesn't yet acknowledge the core power of sexual connection: its ability to transform our lives.

The national conversation about sex trivializes women's most meaningful experiences. Sexual slang reduces us to body parts. The just-say-no language of sexual morality offers too many "shoulds" and "oughts." The clinical language of sexual science shrinks sex to what can be counted or measured—pulses, spasms, hormone levels, goals. In some ways, the language of spiritual experience comes closest to expressing the fullness of our sexual response, for it is the language of connection and ecstasy. I've heard women describe their most joyous sex as "bliss," "a joining of hearts," "a revelation," "a gift from God."

My goal in this book is to expand how we think and talk about sex—by offering information from thousands of women and suggesting how their experiences might broaden sexual meanings and language for all of us.

The Varieties of Sexual Experience

The core information in this book is based on results of a nationwide survey I conducted on integrating sexuality and spirituality—known as the ISIS survey, for short. I received 3,810 responses, making ISIS one of the largest American scientific sex surveys. Most of the ISIS respondents were women. Their ages span seven decades, from late teens into their eighties. These women are diverse in other ways too, including race, religion, education, politics, work, geographic location, sexual attitudes, and the kinds of partners they choose.

The ISIS survey asked respondents how they experience sex and what sex means in their lives. Extraordinarily, this was the first (and so far only) nationwide sex survey to ask these kinds of questions in any depth. Other surveys have asked how many partners you've had, how old you were when you first menstruated, how often you masturbate, have intercourse, and achieve orgasm. We can count and measure all these data, and they help us understand the physiology of sex. But they don't move us toward understanding the deeper purpose of sex in our lives or the power sex has to change our minds, our relationships, and our bodies.

The ISIS survey responses are unique in sexual science. Respondents wrote almost 1,500 letters describing the varieties of their sexual experience. These are remarkable documents, spontaneous, moving, often surprising. They are the first to confirm from women all over the country that there's far more to sex than mainstream experts have led us to believe. They delve into the mysteries of sexual connection—how to open up our hearts and souls, how to let our partners know what we most deeply want, how to keep from being overwhelmed by so much feeling, so much trust, so much light. Their collective story challenges fifty years of performance-oriented norms established by other major sex surveys, from the 1953 *Kinsey Report* to the 1976 *Hite Report* to the 1994 *Social Organization of Sexuality*. The generous spirits of these ISIS women shine on every page of this book.

The Heart and Soul of Sex is based on scientific research, but it's also based on what I've learned in my life—as a clinician since 1974, and as a woman on this planet since well before that (I was thirteen when the first *Kinsey Report* was published). After all these years I know at a deeply personal level that sexual energy permeates our lives from the very beginning. From nursing my babies I've seen how closely pleasure is linked to our first stirrings of life-force—our infant instincts to nuzzle and suck. Nobody's charted when our sexual energy ends, but I was once privileged to witness its glow in a dear person who was only hours from death. His wife had put on a CD of dance tunes they'd loved and he began to move—first a finger then a shoulder. He was dancing! And he was inviting her to join him. She crawled in bed with him and they danced into the night, hearts touching, until he left his body.

The truth is, our sexual energy is always with us, whether or not we choose to act on it in a genital way. It's not just about intercourse and orgasm. It's about receptiveness and movement. It's about our most profound emotions and how we reach out to touch others. It's about how we think and feel and love. It affects every aspect of our lives and it's potentially there until we cease to inhabit this planet. As an ISIS woman wisely said, "Sex isn't everything, but it is a *part* of everything."

USING THIS BOOK AS A GUIDE

The chapters in this book weave together a story about sex that's never been told before in quite this way. The themes come directly from the experience of contemporary women—the thousands who answered the ISIS survey, and thousands more who have attended my lectures, workshops, and therapy sessions over the years. They illustrate the depth and breadth of our sexual responses—from what I call skin hunger to emotional flow to cosmic connection. They acknowledge that sex can be a wellspring of our highest human values. They validate the complexity of our sexual journeys and the wisdom they inspire.

The book also reveals some of the roadblocks to integrating sexual energy into our lives. It tells how the selective sex education we receive as girls and women diminishes our sense of what we can expect as lovers, wives, and mothers—creating a sort of "gaslight" syndrome that so gradually deprives us of light we don't recognize we're functioning in the dark. *The Heart and Soul of Sex* spells out ways we can transcend guilt, shame, and good-girls-don't messages to find sexual safety and sacred union. It offers insights into the ravages of sexual violence, abuse, and substance dependencies—how these can wreak havoc on our sexual choices and our ability to give and receive pleasure. From my years as a marriage and family therapist, I know that a crucial part of recovering the ability to love is sexual recovery—reclaiming those shards of your inner self you've jettisoned in the attempt to outrun your demons.

There is guidance and advice in many of these ISIS stories. Not the mechanical kind that tells you how to turn your engine on and keep it running, but practical nonetheless, because there are suggestions and exercises that really do work if you practice them. The aim is not to set a new sexual standard for women. We've already had too many standards set for us—the last thing we need is to bump the bar up any higher. The aim of this book is to affirm what many women are already experiencing, or at least longing for: intense emotional contact and a sense that true eroticism encompasses much more than intercourse or orgasm or pleasing your partner at the expense of yourself.

In these stories the paths to sexual satisfaction connect physical sensation with spiritual energies such as love, compassion, commitment, empathy, and reverence for life. The intent is to help you discover which paths lead away from your center and which lead you home to yourself.

Part One, "The ISIS Connection," invites you on a journey of discovery. In these eleven chapters you'll travel through a broad new landscape of sexual health and meaning. You'll learn about the ISIS research. You'll be introduced to the ISIS Wheel, a user-friendly model that helps you become aware of the many aspects of your sexual experience—physical, mental, emotional, and spiritual. You'll hear how other women have been able to move beyond old, limiting beliefs about desire and performance to find deep sexual wisdom that's opened their minds and transformed their lives. You'll also learn about a breakthrough in sex research: how contemporary brain studies reveal that all of us have the capacity for sexual responses that are widely multidimensional. This is evidence-based support for the ISIS model of sexual experience.

Part Two, "Paths to the Heart and Soul of Sex," invites you to incorporate these ISIS discoveries into your own life. Here are eight chapters you can use as your personal coach. They can help you move toward more meaningful, satisfying sex even if you have a history of disappointment and abuse. You'll learn about the chakra system to help you open your own flow of sexual energy, and about Tantric techniques to help you connect physical sex with your spiritual values. Steps and strategies in this section include guided imagery; intensive journaling; communication exercises; role-playing; values clarification; affirmations; guidelines for creating sexual ceremony; and playful suggestions for increasing your sensuality, empathy, and spiritual sensitivity.

At the end of the book you'll find the original ISIS questionnaire on integrating sexuality and spirituality so you can see how you might answer these questions—and what your answers have to teach you. There are also suggested readings, counseling resources, and websites that enable you to look beyond this book for information and support. And beyond this book, another book based on the ISIS findings is in the works, one that explores how our relationships impact our sexual experience—as well as more closely examining the issues of sexual desire.

However you decide to use this book, may pleasure and wisdom guide your journey, and may sex touch the depths of your heart and soul.

PART ONE

THE ISIS
CONNECTION

CHAPTER ONE

BROADENING OUR VISION OF SEX

"Isn't there more to sex than this?" This is what nearly every woman coming into my therapy office really wants to know. Whatever her presenting problem, there's an ultimate longing for connection and meaning in sexual experience—for more than intercourse, more than genital foreplay, more than "Was it good for you?"

But in this culture it's difficult for most of us to think about sex in a meaningful way, let alone talk about what we truly want. Our national conversation about sex is mostly limited to performance issues such as intercourse, orgasm, scoring, and who does what with whom how many times a week. Many women feel left out of these conversations. Partly this is because of the just-say-no messages and double messages we receive as girls and women:

"Good girls *don't*."
"Sex is dirty—save it for the one you love."

Messages like these can be especially confusing because explicit sexual images are everywhere in today's media culture, urging us to excitement and romance—and to buy the products that will get us there. These kinds of images lead to more double messages:

"Good girls *don't*—but why can't you put out like that babe on MTV?"

"You don't want sex all the time? Go get a doctor's prescription that will make you hot and horny."

"But don't enjoy yourself *too much*, because there are some nasty names out there for women who love sex." (You can probably come up with at least three of these without even stopping to think.)

As this book progresses, we'll discuss how these kinds of messages got here and why they stay around to haunt us. Sometimes it seems as if the vast ocean of all that women want has to shrink to a puddle to fit today's norms and standards. Men are deluged with their own set of sexual messages and are stymied by cultural norms about how "real men" are supposed act and feel. But when it comes to the topics of sexual desire and performance, women are consistently viewed as not measuring up. Even in these postmodern times women are still considered to be the second sex—a term coined by Simone de Beauvoir back in the repressive 1950s.

WHAT SCIENCE SAYS ABOUT WOMEN'S SEXUAL RESPONSE

Most established sex research has found women to be less sexually interested and less functional than men. But this research has failed to take into account what most women find most deeply satisfying and significant about sex—feelings of overall body pleasure and many other intangibles of sexual experience: passionate connection with our partners, acceptance, release, beauty, and the sense of ongoing personal power when all of these are present.

The most influential model of human sexual response was developed in the mid 1960s by sex researchers William Masters and Virginia Johnson. The Masters-and-Johnson sexual response cycle defines our experience of sex strictly in terms of physiology and performance. It progresses through stages of *arousal* (increased heart rate, blood pressure, muscle tension, and genital engorgement), *plateau* (continued sexual tension), *orgasm* (vaginal and uterine spasms and other releases of sexual tension), and *resolution* (return to the pre-aroused state—when you roll over on your side and go to sleep).

This sexual response cycle has become the gold standard for the diagnosis of sexual problems—and this could have implications for your life. For instance, if your experience of sex departs from this cycle, if you don't easily glide through all these stages and achieve orgasm and even multiple orgasms, you're likely to be labeled "dysfunctional" by your partner, your doctor, and most importantly yourself. Yet how could all of us possibly fit into this model? And where are the emotional and spiritual aspects of sexuality women consistently describe as most important and fulfilling? This medical model omits these crucial aspects of our sexuality and our lives.

If you want to familiarize yourself with the research, I invite you to read Masters and Johnson's *Human Sexual Response* (1966) and also Helen Singer Kaplan's *Disorders of Sexual Desire* (1979), the book that added the phase of sexual desire to the physiologic model of sexual response. Kaplan's work provides the basis for much of our present medicalization of sexual desire, with its focus on neurotransmitters and hormone levels—instead of focusing on asking women what they want.

Sex survey research also tends to reinforce the notion that women lack sexual interest and ability. Like the laboratory study above, most sex surveys focus on performance, not feelings, as the measure of sexual health. A prime example is the University of Chicago's 1994 survey on sexual behavior, where so many women indicated sexual "dissatisfaction" that a follow-up survey was conducted. Some fifteen hundred women were asked if they'd experienced any one of seven sexual problems during the previous year. All of these problems were related to intercourse, and answering "yes" to just one of these characterized a woman as "dysfunctional." From this study has come the stunning statistic that *43 percent of American women are sexually dysfunctional.*

The big problem with this 43-percent figure is that it's been taken as representative of all women and used as evidence that female sexual dysfunction is widespread in this country. I see "43 percent" quoted in scientific journals, in ads for sexual enhancement products, even on *Oprah.*

Again, I invite you to read the original research by Edward Laumann and colleagues: *The Social Organization of Sexuality* (1994) and its 1999 follow-up study by Laumann and colleagues in the *Journal of the American Medical Association*. For a compelling way to think about "43 percent" in the larger frame of women's lives, see the Medscape article by Karen Hicks: "Women's Sexual Problems—A Guide to Integrating the New View Approach."

But these studies are just the tip of the iceberg. In the last hundred years almost 750 sex surveys and countless other studies have been conducted on sexual response. These invariably define sex in terms of intercourse and/or orgasm—and almost none of them asks for details about how women feel and what sex means to them. The point is, when our notions of sex are based on research that leaves out our emotions and meanings and the context of our lives, how can we know the real difference between function and dysfunction, satisfaction and dissatisfaction, or what those labels actually mean?

One result of all this surfaces in my sex therapy practice. I find that many women can't even begin to articulate what deep and lasting sexual pleasure might mean for them. They can only name their sexual problems. "Low libido" is a hot-button issue these days, and pharmaceutical companies are scrambling to create a cream or patch or pill that will make women feel as juicy as teenagers and, hopefully, mad with desire.

But—and this is one of the questions too many researchers fail to ask—mad with desire for what? For Friday-night intercourse with a husband who doesn't know how to make eye contact? For a lover who's more concerned with technique than with what you feel? Sultry lovemaking at the tail end of working two jobs and caring for three kids? A harassed mother told me she didn't have enough time to shave both of her legs during the same shower, let alone imagine seducing her partner. Another woman admitted she was so disengaged that she watched the late show on her bedside TV while her husband mounted her. And I've heard too many women weep over the cruel truth that even the most loving sexual touch can restimulate memories of sexual abuse. This kind of exasperation, exhaustion, and disaffection can't be cured by a patch or a pill or even a hot new technique.

THE GOOD NEWS ABOUT
WOMEN'S SEXUALITY

These problems may sound daunting, but take heart. There's a whole other story of women's sexuality waiting to be told, a positive story filled with potential. *The Heart and Soul of Sex* will show you ways you can find the "more" so many women crave—the love, passion, closeness, empathy, and respect; the mutual caring and pleasure; the sense of renewed energy; the sense of connectedness to your partner (if you have one), and most importantly to yourself.

The first step to these kinds of "more" begins with broadening your vision—looking beyond performance definitions of sex to all that sexual relationship can be. Intercourse and orgasm may be the way sex has been defined for us—but they're only a small part of being a sexual person. Women who've talked with me want to feel good inside as well as outside. They want love and acceptance. They want their partners to flow with them like water. They want to let go, really let go, even if just for once in their lives.

More women than you might think are hovering at the edge of their inhibitions and fears, ready to open up to intimate connections of body, mind, heart, and spirit. "Sometimes I feel like a landslide about to happen," one woman confided to me. Throughout this book you'll be hearing inspiring stories and reflections from women who are exploring the infinite varieties of sexual relationship.

Who are these women? In many ways they're probably like you (you'll learn more about them in the next chapter). You'll see that they have much to teach about how we can move from negative sexual experiences to positive ones. Their stories demonstrate that sex can be much more than we've been told, that our sexual experience can touch our souls, even transform our lives.

The idea of broadening your vision of sex may seem new and exciting—or it may seem scary or even impossible. I ask you for a leap of faith. Allow yourself to trust the women in this book as I've trusted them. Let them take you by the hand and show you some of the paths they've discovered that lead them to pleasure and wholeness, and sometimes to quantum life changes along the way.

A JOURNEY OF TRANSFORMATION

What began to broaden my own view of sex was a letter from a researcher colleague in Georgia. In 1994 she sent me a story about her first big love relationship, and it scrambled my notions of how women experience sexual intimacy. "It was like being touched by God," she wrote. "Not that my partner was God, but that the intensity of our lovemaking was proof that God existed, that only God could have created anything so powerful and positive."

In one sense, her words came as no surprise, for I'd heard so many women describe mountaintop experiences—when the earth moved and time stood still. And I'd experienced those moments too. In fact this kind of extraordinary sexual connection has sparked some of my own important choices—from making a life commitment with my beloved partner to launching a career as a sex therapist and researcher. Yet this colleague was voicing a truth I'd never heard articulated so succinctly: that sex—even the most intensely physical sex—may be far more spiritual than most of us have dared imagine.

Her letter arrived while I was on the road promoting the first edition of *Women Who Love Sex,* a book I'd written to broaden people's understanding of how women experience sexual health and pleasure. In nearly every audience someone raised a hand to comment, "The women in your book are talking about sex, but they're also talking about spirituality!"

How astonishing it was to hear those two words in the same sentence. Our culture carefully separates our sexual experience from our spiritual experience. Our moral and religious traditions tend to teach us that too much pleasure pollutes the spirit. We're taught to think in terms of black-and-white opposites and contradictions—yes/no, good/bad, old/young, gay/straight, Mars/Venus. And of course sex/spirit.

Yet here I was, meeting women all over the country who were saying something different. I began asking them how they connected sexual pleasure with what they felt was most sacred and holy—loving their partners; communing with nature; worshipping God, Goddess, or other heavenly beings. Everyone seemed to have a story. Some spoke of emotional and spiritual ecstasy. Some described profound healing that came from connecting sex and spirit, even after histories of sexual abuse. Through all their stories, the message ran clear: "good girls" *can* love sex—and many of them do. And all these women's stories contained a central truth: that spirit is a part of sex, not apart from it.

This collective message so strongly reinforced my colleague's letter that I made a decision that was to alter my life. I began in earnest to explore the connections between sexuality and spirituality. Almost immediately it struck me that I'd spent over two decades learning all I could about sex and sexual relationships—I'd acquired a doctorate in sexology, I'd treated clients, taught classes, written books, received grants and awards. But I had no consistent spiritual practice, and that felt like a great void. I'd grown up in a family that belonged to no religion (unless it counts that they religiously kept the cocktail hour). Even as a child I yearned to connect with something "out there," but I didn't know what it was or where to look. Now here was the opportunity handed to me on a platter. I realized it was time to pay attention to where the universe was already leading me and stay open to what would unfold.

As soon as I made this decision, a series of remarkable teachers appeared—they say this happens when the student is ready. The story of these encounters could probably fill another book. But for purposes here, I plunged deeply into the earth-honoring practice of Andean shamanism. Looking back, this was a natural choice, as my lineage is Peruvian on my father's side, and at one level it felt like a way to contact ancestors I'd never known. At another level, this practice opened up new ways to understand the subtle connections between physical, emotional, mental, and spiritual energy—and how these connections relate to our sexuality. This understanding underlies the concept of the ISIS Wheel that you will meet in chapter 4.

In the course of these spiritual explorations, I also became aware of the complex ways women have experienced sexual energy over the ages. I saw that the rich connections between women, sex, and spirit trace back to the most ancient of cultures. These connections survive in stunning images today—in sculptures of fertility goddesses giving birth to the sun, moon, and stars; in labyrinths that wind into the womb of the Great Mother; and, on every continent, yoni caves shaped like vulvas—that's right, openings in the bedrock that look exactly like the folds of women's vaginas and birth canals, huge, beautiful, and quite astounding. These caves have been worshipped since time immemorial. I learned that the entry into women's sexual mysteries has always been connected with the entry into the deepest mysteries of the planet.

Living in our contemporary American culture, I began to feel as if we are inhabiting a sexual Dark Age. Sex is treated as more of an embarrassment than a blessing. Too often we express sex as a joke, a dirty word, a body part shouted in anger, or a personal put-down such as "slut" or "faggot." Too often sex is used as a form of social control rather than a way of connecting deeply with one another.

There's also a curious paradox. While all manner of sexual activity is available on your TV and over the Internet, real-life sex is supposed to hide behind closed doors. Shhh! Don't talk about it! This holds true even when you're openly in love and solidly joined in a lifelong relationship. Hardly ever do we hear sex discussed as a multidimensional whole, in all its cultural, physical, emotional, relational, meaningful, developmental, healing, lusty, transformational aspects. The idea that sex can assume mystical proportions as a life-altering experience is not yet part of our national conversation. There's no common definition of positive sexuality that applies to the whole woman in the context of her life's complexities. To most of the world the word "sex" still means "intercourse." That is, it means performance.

There's an inherent problem with the performance definition of sex. It tends to bypass our feelings and meanings. It bypasses our deep connections with the rhythms of the planet. It perpetuates a stereotype that keeps many women locked into a kind of cultural missionary position, man on top. Not a position of safety for most women—or pleasure, either. Rather, it's a position that encourages some women to fake orgasm. Far more devastatingly, it encourages us to fake intimacy with our partners. And when we do that, we compromise our honesty with ourselves.

All of this led me to understand that the next challenge in promoting the well-being of women—and men, too—was to broaden the definition of sex. I wondered what would happen if women had the opportunity to describe the full scope of their sexual experience—pleasures, empowerments, and divine revelations, as well as complaints and disasters.

Extraordinarily, I found that no one had yet conducted a national survey that investigated the spiritual dimensions of our everyday sexual experiences. Even the most highly respected sex surveys had made no serious attempt to explore the deeper, personal meanings of sex. These included the massive *Kinsey Reports* of 1948 (on male sexual behavior) and 1953 (on female sexual behavior), as well as the 1994 survey cited earlier, and the hundreds of surveys in between.

The truth is, these surveys rarely touched on the emotional issues such as sensitivity, love, commitment, intimacy, empathy, and self-esteem. Instead they focused on numbers of partners and frequencies of intercourse. They established orgasm as the primary indicator of sexual health, and coital activity as the primary indicator of sexual interest. Thus the immense subject of our sexual attitudes and behavior was being determined by focus on a few body parts. It seemed to me like the proverbial blind men trying to describe an elephant. Consistently, the elephant called human sexuality was being portrayed as possessing enormous genitals but very little heart, mind, or capacity for complexity.

This troubled me deeply because what's left out are exactly the issues women were bringing into my therapy sessions and workshops—all those women who want "more." And a scary truth was beginning to filter into my consciousness: *Sex survey research has been systematically shortchanging all of those women (and plenty of men, too) by asking the wrong questions.*

I was certain that with new questions would come different conclusions, and that a more positive sexual scenario would unfold. I knew that a vast and inclusive story about our sexual response waited to be told, one that transcends intercourse, orgasm, "scoring," and gender stereotypes. I also knew that the time was ripe. Americans are fascinated by sex. And in recent years there's been a steady gush of interest in spiritual consciousness, mind-body health, and spiritual practices. Why not explore spirituality as an integral factor in sexual response and sexual relationships? Feeling somewhat like a pioneer venturing into the wilderness, I set out to create a survey I hoped could begin to bring the story of women's sexuality into the twenty-first century.

CHAPTER TWO

THE ISIS SURVEY
IS BORN

THE SURVEY I CREATED is titled "Integrating Sexuality and Spirituality." It investigates sexuality, love, relationship, commitment, religion, spirituality, intimacy, safety, empathy, and communication. Not until I was seeking a shorthand for this book did the acronym "ISIS" appear. Quite magically, this also happens to be the name of the Egyptian goddess, the most powerful and widely worshipped deity in human history—for over three thousand years. Her story so curiously parallels this project that I want to introduce her here.

Isis, the Great Cosmic Mother, is known as the Goddess of a Thousand Names—among them: Creator of Life, Death, and Regeneration; Queen of Heaven and Earth; Lady of Love and Abundance; Initiator into the Sexual Mysteries. The story goes that her husband, Osiris, was hacked to bits by his power-crazed brother, and his remains were scattered far and wide. Isis wandered the corners of the earth gathering up all the pieces of her husband's body. She was able to find everything except his penis. Undaunted, she created a penis out of clay, breathed Osiris back to life, and conceived his child.

I believe Isis is a wonderfully fitting name to invoke in connection with this survey and this book—whose spirit is to search out the lost pieces of our sexuality and put them back together to create new life.

CREATING AND DISTRIBUTING
THE ISIS SURVEY

Because I conducted the survey as an independent researcher, I could ask any questions I chose. If I'd been an academic, I'd have had to base the questions on earlier surveys. If I'd been funded by an institution, I'd have had to base them on the constraints of the funders. So goes the way of academic research. And so goes any semblance of total objectivity. Sex researchers and other scientists speak about the great value of being objective and nonjudgmental. But if you think about it, all survey research is based on somebody's bias, somebody's idea, somebody's passion, whether it's the researcher's, the institution's, or that of the corporation that provides the funding.

So I decided to let my personal biases blossom. I asked survey respondents how they connected sexuality and spirituality—was it through excitement? honesty? laughter? commitment? caring for others? and so forth. I asked the question "In a moment of sexual ecstasy have you ever had a sense of experiencing God?" I noted that sexual romance and religious worship have many kinds of symbols and rituals in common, such as candles, incense, flowers, wine, and I asked respondents to check all of these that they associated with both sexuality and spirituality.

These questions and many more came directly from issues raised by women—the clients and colleagues who'd so openly trusted me over the years with their life stories. Not that I feel men's issues are unimportant. Rather, I saw that women needed to tell this particular story because our voices are so vastly underrepresented in sex research. Women need an opportunity to let the world know what we want as well as what we don't want. I knew women's complaints and dysfunctions were already amply documented by other sex surveys, the ones that asked about frequencies (how many times you do what with whom) but not how you feel about it or what it means to you.

ISIS wasn't an easy survey to create, because the issues it tackles are so unusual to sex surveys. Plus, they tap directly into a deep cultural taboo: the national terror of endowing our sensual, sexual pleasures with any measure of spiritual value. One woman who volunteered for an original pilot group phrased the problem vividly. "I can fill out the sex part," she said, "but the spirituality part is really scary. My grandmother was an Italian Catholic, and I can feel her turning over in her grave right now at the thought of bringing these two ideas together."

I consulted a dozen colleagues to help me create a questionnaire that was not only scientific but also engaging enough—and safe enough—for people to answer. Then there was another choice to make. How would I find people to answer my survey? Should this be a random sample? Random sampling means that researchers place a grid over a map and contact unsuspecting folk who represent certain areas. This is the kind of survey sampling contemporary science likes because it's supposed to reach people who have no biases about your subject. Which is fine if your subject is laundry soap. But everybody has biases about sex, no matter where they live. Besides, I knew random sampling in sex research has too often misrepresented women. It's portrayed them as less interested, less satisfied, and more dysfunctional than men—and experience has led me to doubt the truth of that. Also, ISIS was to be an exploratory survey. Nobody had ever asked these particular questions before. I wanted to find people who were likely to have connected sex and spirit in their own lives, because I knew they were most likely to offer informative, interesting answers. A special population to be sure, but one that could provide a baseline for other researchers to build upon.

So I chose to use another survey method: a sample of convenience. In my case that meant I handed the printed questionnaire to almost everyone I was in contact with in the last half of 1997 and asked if they'd be willing to fill out the survey. Some of them then asked to distribute the survey to their colleagues and students, and so it went. Over a thousand completed surveys came back to me—from students, nurses, family therapists, clergy, and people in a variety of sexual lifestyles. To elicit a variety of views, I'd particularly sought to contact people from groups that are known to have opposing ideas about both sexuality and spirituality. These groups included Catholic clergy and pro-choice activists, male sex offenders and female abuse survivors, fundamentalist Christians and lesbian women.

Finding respondents in this way doesn't mean the survey results are less accurate than they might have been by random sampling. But it does mean the results apply only to those people who answered the survey, not to everyone in America, or the world, or the universe. The downside is that critics can argue that these respondents selected themselves, so their opinions may not reflect what the rest of the world thinks and feels. There's an upside, too. It means that you, the reader, don't have to take what the respondents say as carved-in-stone imperatives. You're totally free to decide whether or not what all these ISIS respondents said actually applies to your sexual experience and your life.

Once I started distributing the questionnaire, the process snowballed in a major way. Soon two national magazines asked to reprint the questionnaire for their readers to fill out. "Integrating Sexuality and Spirituality" appeared in the January–February 1998 issue of *New Age* magazine (now titled *Body and Soul*) and in the July 1998 issue of *New Woman*. Readers of these magazines accounted for almost three thousand more completed surveys.

News of the project even got to Oprah Winfrey—thanks to my long-time supporter Dr. Christiane Northrup. In May 2000 I appeared on the *Oprah* show to talk about my research. When the producer called me out of the blue, my first words were, "Thanks, but no thanks—I don't want to be on television!" (Well, I was just beginning to analyze all the survey results—what would I say? And even more anxiety-provoking, what was I going to wear?) Joan Oliver, my *New Age* editor, howled with glee when I told her this story—"You're the only person alive who's ever turned down a chance to be on *Oprah!*" But in the end, the producer patiently explained that Oprah wanted me to help counteract all the hype about Viagra and testosterone. I leaped to the challenge—and as it turned out, the delight. When Oprah cast her gaze on me and we began to talk before the cameras, her energy opened and I could feel her scoop my words into her being and translate them for her audience. She was engagingly present, she was filled with spirit, she was sexy, she was queen of her universe. Clearly, this ISIS project had led me into the presence of a modern-day goddess.

WHO ANSWERED THE ISIS SURVEY?

When I started the project, I'd expected to hear from a couple hundred people. But by the time the dust cleared, nearly four thousand had responded. Completed surveys poured in by fax and mail from every state in the United States and from two Canadian provinces (this was just before so many of us began communicating by e-mail). More than three thousand responses came from women, and a surprising 684 men answered the survey as well, along with 11 responses from people who identified themselves as transgendered. The respondents included churchgoers and atheists, conservatives and liberals, pro-choice and anti-abortion advocates. They worked as teachers, physicians, nurses, clergy, homemakers, students, artists, office personnel, and manual laborers. They also revealed identities less likely to be discussed in everyday conversation: they were lesbians, gay men, bisexuals, and transgendered individuals; sexual abuse survivors and sex offenders; addicts and recovering addicts; survivors of religious cults; prisoners; sex industry workers; and cross-dressers. They were single, widowed, divorced. They were partnered in relationships they variously described as ecstatic unions, sexless marriages, clandestine affairs, or polyamorous partnerships, that is, sexual intimacy with more than one ongoing partner.

Remarkably, 1,465 of these respondents sent letters describing their experiences. Many more jotted informal notes in the margins of the survey itself. Their stories and jottings express themes that are universal to women's sexual well-being: the need for self-esteem; the yearning for human touch, nurturing, intimacy, and love; the desire for meaning and continuity; and joy in the delicious flow of connecting sex and spirit.

Even as teetering piles of these questionnaires and letters threatened to take over my office and living space, I was overwhelmed with their significance. For one thing, I was awed that the extraordinary number of responses was placing the ISIS survey among the large scientific sex surveys of North America. But the significance of these ISIS responses far supersedes their numbers. They're uniquely valuable because they're the first to broaden our vision of sexual experience beyond physiology and performance.

Key ISIS Findings and What They Mean for Women

The ISIS findings document some essential facts of sexual experience that cannot be measured or proved in any quantifiable way. These are the emotional and spiritual subtleties that engage our minds, hearts, and spirits as well as our bodies. The ISIS findings confirm that sex can be a path to spiritual awakening. They also show that spiritual development can lead to sexual awakening at any age. They offer new insights about relationship, life-span issues, religious messages, abuse, and healing. They challenge some conventional notions of sexual response, sexual relationship, and sexual healing.

Sexual response is multidimensional

The first and most fundamental finding of the ISIS survey is that sex is more than just a physical experience. ISIS women say sex touches their minds and hearts as well as their bodies. Some say that sexual experience also touches their souls. For these women sex can be an entry into the realm of revelation and grace—what a fifty-three-year-old graphic artist describes as "the door to greater love, a greater sense of awe, and greater dimensions of spiritual experience." Other women speak of sexual energy opening up to a universe of vibrant light and color, spontaneous healing, memories of prior lifetimes, and direct encounters with divinity—God, Goddess, and other benevolent beings.

In the chapters that follow we'll see how these many realities of sexual experience unfold into a powerful new vision of what sex can mean for women—and how you can discover this vision for yourself. Meanwhile, below are some numbers that reflect how ISIS women regard their sexual responses as more than physical.

What stands out for me here is that so many ISIS women affirm a truth that's outside of the common conversation about sex. Namely that sexual experience involves much more than intercourse, more than genital stimulation, more than arousal or orgasm or even physical attraction. These women are broadening our definitions of what it means to be sexual. As you

ISIS Women by the Numbers

In What Ways Is Sex More than Physical?

86% say sex also involves love, romance, and mystical union

79% say sex releases their emotional tension

75% say sex intensifies their inner vitality

67% say sex needs to be spiritual to be satisfying

59% say their spiritual beliefs open them to risk deeper intimacy

47% say they've experienced God during sexual ecstasy

45% say they've experienced sexual energy during spiritual ecstasy

can see from the numbers above, most ISIS women agree that emotional feelings and spiritual meanings are crucial to sexual experience and satisfaction. Nearly half of these women say they find that physical sex is a direct path to God—and that spirituality can be a path to physical pleasure.

How do these ISIS women compare with the rest of the world's women? There's no way of knowing. The ISIS responses are unique because questions about sex and spirit have never been systematically researched on a large scale before. What's important is how these women's perceptions may help you think about your own sexual responses and your own life, so that you understand what's true for you. It may be that you've never thought about questions like these—about 15 percent of ISIS respondents said they'd never thought of spirituality as a part of sex before they answered the survey. So take heart. Read on. And embark on a journey of discovery.

Erotic satisfaction is primarily experienced in the context of relationship

This finding focuses on women in all kinds of relationships—marriages, affairs, lifelong loves, one-night stands, partnerships with men and with women. Here we find one of the most consistent themes of the ISIS survey: love between partners is a powerful catalyst for sex that is meaningful and satisfying. A fifty-year-old physical therapist from Bozeman, Montana, puts it succinctly: "I don't have sex—I make love! Big difference. Sex between lovers creates a miracle of intimacy." In fact, nearly nine of every ten ISIS women say love is essential to their sexual satisfaction. In the course of this book women talk about many factors that contribute to satisfaction in their sexual relationships. Here are a few numbers to consider before you read their stories:

ISIS Women by the Numbers

What Aspects of Relationship Deepen Sexual Satisfaction?

86% say love and acceptance
83% say being in love
81% say sharing deep feelings
80% say honesty
73% say laughing together
63% say caring for others
63% say letting go of control
61% say feeling safe

Several things stand out for me as I think about these numbers. One is that so many women equate sexual satisfaction with love and acceptance. Not a surprise perhaps, but notice that an almost equal number of women mention that honesty and sharing deep feelings are essential to opening their erotic sensibilities. This says to me that sex may be most meaningful when you're most open with one another about what you think, feel, and know. It also says that emotional intimacy makes it possible to explore the deeper dimensions of physical sex.

Nearly two-thirds of these ISIS women say caring for others is an essential ingredient for sexual satisfaction. I think this number might have been much higher if it had not been paired with "caring for self" (meaning that respondents had to make a choice between whether sexual satisfaction was linked to nurturing themselves or others). This is one of the pesky problems with survey design that may not show up until it's too late to change. Hopefully future researchers will correct this error by separating these questions—important because the capacity to care deeply for both yourself and your partner are so crucial to women's sexual satisfaction and to fully relational sex.

ISIS numbers also suggest that partners who laugh together may feel safe enough to let go of social controls—the inhibiting kind that say women should be "good girls" and also dutiful sex partners. This dictum is a classic double message of course, one that immobilizes many a woman before the blush is off her wedding vows. But clearly these ISIS women say they enjoy both physical sex and spiritual "goodness." Still, the researcher in me wonders: How might these laughing, caring, occasionally mystical women answer a sex survey that asks only about intercourse, orgasm, and number of partners? Might some of these women score low to middling on these questions and land in the vast statistical pool of American women that researchers say just don't like sex? Notice how the whole sexual picture becomes brighter for women when they respond to questions about the meanings of sexual relationship instead of the frequencies of sexual intercourse. For some, it's as if they've been blown out of Kansas and into Oz.

Connecting sexuality and spirituality promotes personal and cultural healing

The healing connection is where ISIS women are at their most innovative and courageous. Especially so considering that many of them experienced sexual abuse—27 percent as children and 15 percent as adults (just two percentage points higher than the national average, according to the 2000 U.S. Census). ISIS women write that connecting sex and spirit expands their sense of self, love, creativity, well-being, altruism, and union with a higher power. Some say they've actually used their old negative experiences as paths to joy in their present relationships. A thirty-four-year-old Nevada psychologist says she realized the "gift" of being molested once she was able to clear the anger, shame, and hatred she carried. In her words, coming to terms with these "forced me to love my body and soul for its life force, pleasure, creativity, and power."

This finding about sexual healing has an optimistic and far-reaching message: Integrating sexuality and spirituality is a means of fully embracing not only ourselves and one another but also the planet. It's in this healing journey that we learn to distinguish between pleasure and pain, empathy and control, love and hate, caring and neglect, giving and taking, justice and brute violence.

The ISIS bottom line is that our most intimate relationships form a template for all our relationships—with ourselves, our partners, our community, our environment, and with the world of spirit and divinity. Women offer thought-provoking images of nonviolence to counteract the domestic abuse, gay-bashing, random shootings, and strategic bombings that have become our daily media fare. In the words of a research fellow from Maryland, integrating sex and spirit can become "an awesome tool for transcending the mundane and communicating with the source of all power and life."

As I lived and worked with the thousands of survey responses that poured in, I felt enormous gratitude toward all the individuals who'd braved convention to answer these questions, who'd perhaps overridden their traditional biases and tuned in to truths that ventured far beyond how the culture defines sexual experience. I vowed that I'd honor their offerings with the care and reverence they deserved. And since so many respondents expressed a wish that their experiences be used to help others, I committed myself to doing all I could to bring their news to the largest possible audience. Attending to these vows meant plunging back into academic study for three years before I felt I could analyze the data in the most responsible way. Then I needed another couple of years to recover from the constraints of academic discourse and begin to present the ISIS findings in user-friendly prose.

In the following chapters I'll show how these ISIS findings can help broaden the language we use to describe and define sex, and I'll explore many avenues you can use for your own health, growth, and healing. As Oprah herself suggested when I appeared on her show, these responses pose the possibility that sex, even the wham-bam variety, may be the door to ineffable grace.

CHAPTER THREE

OPENING THE CIRCLE, STARTING YOUR JOURNEY

ISIS WOMEN ASSERT that healthy sexual response is much more than rushing headlong toward a goal of orgasm. I've heard this idea expressed by thousands of clients, colleagues, and women who have attended my lectures and workshops. Still it's been deeply affirming to hear it from even more thousands of survey respondents.

In the ISIS model, sexual experience encompasses many realities—sensual feelings, emotional passions, and spiritual meanings. The ISIS model allows for all sorts of individual differences. It encompasses nuances of relationship that may not appear in self-help books. It acknowledges that our sexual experiences are linked to our overall energy and health. And it acknowledges that sexual energy is everywhere—not just in the bedroom behind closed doors.

Since the ISIS model is so much more complex than the performance model, we can't map it with the same simplicity as the physiological models we saw in chapter 1. Nor can we say with the same certainty that it applies to all people at all times. Exploring the breadth and depth of our sexuality means entering uncharted terrain. This is a multidimensional landscape—and there's no way of knowing exactly what kind of weather might blow in once you set out on your journey.

When we think about sex as more than physical, the very word "sexy" can take on new meanings. One of my favorite examples of this occurred when a *Women Who Love Sex* reading group was discussing the "sexiest words" their husbands had ever uttered. An exhausted young mother of four admitted that these words weren't about cliché fantasies, like "You look so great in black lace lingerie," or "Let's you and me take a slow cruise to Bali." They weren't even about love and romance, in the sense of hearts and flowers. They were about empathy—about her equally overworked sweetie understanding exactly what she needed at that moment. His sexiest words? "Tonight I'll do the dishes."

A Gift That Keeps on Giving

The ISIS model also encompasses time and space. Our sexual response begins long before we become physically aroused, and even long before we enter the bedroom. It's informed by our midnight dreams, our daytime activities, and much more. It's informed by our entire life's history—all the way back to our earliest needs and nurturings, pleasures and pains, loves and betrayals. This means that if you've been appropriately adored and cuddled in your early years, you're likely to feel adoringly sexual as an adult, if the circumstances are right. Every cell and synapse remembers those early experiences and feeds positive messages directly into your adult responses to sexual stimulation. By the same token, memories of neglect and abuse can feed fear and even loathing to your here-and-now sexual response.

These messages travel by the neural pathways that have been well described in the mind-body literature. You can find countless examples of the effects of memory—as both destroyer and healer. Psychiatrist Alice Miller is among the many authors who have written movingly of the long-term effects of cruelty to children. Ellen Bass and Laura Davis (*The Courage to Heal*), and Wendy Maltz (*The Sexual Healing Journey*) have written powerful books about how to heal from the devastating effects of sexual abuse. Little is written about the long-term effects of positive sexual experience, though. I'll have to rely on what women have told me in therapy sessions and workshops, and most recently in letters they've written in response to the ISIS survey.

The consensus from ISIS women is that our positive sexual experiences influence us as powerfully as our negative ones do. And they influence us for just as long. The problem is that we don't have permission in this culture to fully explore those positive sexual responses. Women have finally won the right to say no to violence, abuse, and unsafe sex. This is a great victory. But we have work yet to do. It's still not so okay to say yes to pleasure, which is a primary source of our power and beauty and sense of belonging. In terms of mind-blowing, self-affirming, emotionally juicy, transformational sexual experience, the cultural message for us is still a resounding "just say no."

In its fullest and richest form, sexual experience generates a power that flies under the radar of cultural convention. The energy may take on a life of its own. It can overflow your bedroom to influence every aspect of your life—past, present, and future. A delighted colleague once remarked, "I can take it to work with me on the bus the next morning and my whole day feels wonderful." But this kind of whole-person sexual experience can lead to much more than a happy bus ride. Many ISIS women assert that it's changed their minds, literally rewiring how they think about their sexual identities. It's also effected a quantum leap in their belief systems by transporting them to other levels of consciousness, other times and spaces. "A higher place," says a thirty-year-old housewife from Altoona, Pennsylvania. "Another plane of existence," says a fifty-four-year-old counselor from Lowell, Massachusetts. "In the midst of orgasm . . . the presence of God," says a forty-seven-year-old conference coordinator from Louisville, Kentucky.

A fifty-one-year-old antique dealer from San Jose, California, describes this kind of deep sex as changing her entire outlook on life:

This was not growth, this was transformation. I began to learn about and practice unconditional love, and it was magic. My spirituality exploded and enveloped everything. All aspects of my life became a seamless whole, so that there was no separation between spirituality and love, between spirituality and sex, between spirituality and relationship, between spirituality and everyday life. I have begun to see everything with new eyes—nothing is the same. I am like a baby, fresh and new, knowing nothing and having to start all over again. It is difficult to find the words to explain this experience, and to fit it into a questionnaire is utterly impossible.

THE ISIS CIRCLE
An Arena for Change

The ISIS model of sexual experience developed from my workshops for women. The basic form of the model is a circle—an ongoing continuum without an end or a beginning. Women have gathered in circles like this from time immemorial to pound corn, share news, and pass on their stories and secrets.

I invite you to enter just such a circle now. Even though you're probably alone reading this book, you can enter into a circle of women through your imagination.

Gathering in this circle with other women, we bring our bodies together to create a space in the center. This is not an empty space, but a space that vibrates with potential. A space that invites open sharing and heart-to-heart communication. It's generous enough to hold all of us, no matter what our story is. It becomes a spiritual container for all of us and for our sexual stories.

I introduce our space as secret, in the sense that each woman's story is absolutely confidential. And as sacred, in the sense that every story is honored, held in tenderness and trust. It's through this space, this center, that we can encourage and support each other to move beyond our histories of mixed sexual messages, disappointment, and abuse. Here we can reframe negativity and reveal our own profiles in courage. And we can build on each other's positive stories to open to the deepest mysteries that our sexual energy holds.

I ask each woman to bring two objects to place in the circle as offerings. One object represents an aspect of your sexual story you want to let go of. The other represents an aspect of your sexual story you want to keep. As you read this, I invite you to think about what you might bring to such a gathering, or to a gathering that you might initiate yourself.

What women choose to bring to the circle runs the gamut from sacred items (such as crystals and goddess figures) to childhood teddy bears. A young paralegal flung a tube of brand-name lipstick into the center to symbolize her release from what she called "fashion fascism." The woman to her right later asked if she could please take that lipstick home to help her upgrade her own self-image—and she did. A family physician brought a glittery red spike-heeled shoe that symbolized her days of bar-hopping and risky one-night partners. We burned it in a ceremonial fire that night.

All the offerings that come from our experience are gifts of instruction. What women place in the center become agents of change, medicine for healing old wounds and repatriating lost aspects of our selves. We never know from whom the healing will come or on whom it will land. As each woman places her offerings and speaks about them, we are co-creating an organic altar that contains all of our stories, all the group's energy. This is a blueprint for magic, a mandala of change. I have been humbled by the learning and healing I've witnessed in these circles. I've been humbled by my own learning and healing.

In one circle, a woman offered her wedding ring. She told us that her husband had committed suicide more than a year before, on Valentine's Day, and that she was finally ready to become a sexual being again—but she didn't know where to start. That weekend I could feel her struggle in my own body and I felt it was only right to share my own relationship with suicide—that of my mother, on Mother's Day, when I was twenty-two. I shared that I'd carried the grief in my body for decades. That I felt in shock and sexually dead until after my children were born, as if their births had somehow lifted the curse and awakened me.

We cried. And the group cried with us. Each woman mourned a precious piece of her own sexual being that she had lost or had had taken from her. We were in resonance with the spiritual core of our sexual beings. We navigated the river of our collective grief as if we were on a journey into the unseen world. In retrospect it was like the classic canoe ride of shamanic cultures where the mourners paddle in synchrony to the land of the dead and return reborn to life.

The important concept here is that we did return to life. We brought ourselves back home to that magical space in the center of our circle where we drank in the healing energy. Then we went outside and played in the spring sunshine, running with open arms like children let out for recess.

INVITATION TO JUMP
A Meditation

Here is the kind of interactive meditation I use to open each new circle. This one begins with a Native American saying. Its origins are lost in the mists of time, but it expresses a view that's essential for our time and place, for our survival and happiness.

> As you go the way of your life
> you will come to a great chasm.
> Jump! It is not as wide as you think.

In our culture today there's a great chasm between body and soul, sex and spirit. This reflects the divide-and-conquer dualism of the last millennia—divisions between men and women, straight and gay, black and white, child and adult, love and hate, function and dysfunction, winning and losing, even war and peace.

You're welcome to stop and reflect here on whatever chasms you may be facing in your own sexual experience. Perhaps you have doubts or fears. You may feel angry or shut down. You may feel a disconnect between what you want and what others expect of you.

All of us encounter many chasms in the course of our lifetimes, even in the course of each day. We come together in this circle to create a time out of time—and a space where we can revisit our sexuality in terms of wholeness and continuity and support rather than division and isolation.

This is a new way for most of us to think about our sexual selves because we've been taught to see sex as performance. Or as an either/or proposition. Achieve orgasm or be called dysfunctional. Want what your partner wants or be called names that diminish you—abnormal, frigid, deviant, unnatural, slut, prude.

It can be scary to think outside the box our culture builds around us. Even to think of thinking outside that box. If we do, we might have to give up being "good girls." We might have to give up our dysfunctions. We might have to let go of our compulsion to please others. In the process of changing we might lose our power positions. We might lose our minds— our willingness to make sense out of double standards and separation.

Our lives are full of chasms, choices, impasses, possibilities. How can we get to the other side? Sometimes the only choice is to jump.

So when you're ready, let's jump into exploring the ISIS Wheel. It's the next step on our journey. For some women it's a big step and for others it's not so big after all. It may help you to know that you don't have to make this step alone. Many women will be going along with you in the course of this book.

CHAPTER FOUR

THE ISIS WHEEL

Finding Your Path

THE ISIS WHEEL of Sexual Experience is a graphic way to think about the multidimensional nature of human sexual response. It is central to understanding the ISIS connection—the sexual meeting of our bodies, minds, hearts, and spirits. You can use this wheel to map your own sexual responses. This chapter will help you identify where you might want to begin exploring the ISIS connections in your life.

The idea for the ISIS Wheel came about when I was searching for a coherent way to teach students about the vast scope of the responses to the ISIS survey. I needed a model that was different from the goal-oriented models of sex, such as the Masters-and-Johnson phases of orgasm that isolate our sexual responses from the rest of our lives. (It's also a self-destructing model. You get aroused, you explode into orgasm, and boom, sex is over; get back to your life.)

In my earlier writings I have challenged these physiological models by proposing a continuum of pleasure, orgasm, and ecstasy to reflect the ongoing nature of our positive sexual energy (see the third chapter of *Women Who Love Sex*). But to describe the ISIS information, I needed a new, comprehensive model. It needed to reflect more than the positive effects of our peak sexual experiences. It needed to reflect the widely diverse points of view so many women (and men) have shared with me—not only the peaks but also the valleys and the scary abysses. It needed to be expansive enough to contain the physical, emotional, mental, and spiritual aspects of our sexual response. It needed to be open enough to show how sexual experiences are intimately connected with the rest of our lives.

I thought of my women's circles, like those in the previous chapter, which had generated so much ISIS conversation over the years. And beyond those specific gatherings, I pondered the geometry of the circle itself. The circle is an ancient symbol of communication, a roundtable among equals. It's also an age-old symbol of wholeness. It has no beginning and no end. It's found in spiritual traditions around the world—in spirals and labyrinths, in sacred diagrams from the ornate mandalas of Tibetan Buddhism to Native American medicine wheels to the Andean Mesa tradition that is part of my own spiritual practice.

As I learned more about these sacred wheels and mandalas, I began to understand how they are built upon multiple levels of meaning. Details vary from tradition to tradition, but there are commonalities. They all represent the forces of nature and the elements—air, fire, earth, and water. They are rooted in the four corners of the universe—north, south, east, and west. They represent the celestial and the secular. And always they contain teachings connected with our lives—our carnality and divinity, our humanity, and our hunger for connection, meaning, and transcendence. Working with these sacred diagrams has helped people all over the world move through the dark nights of their souls and into profound states of healing.

I knew the ISIS material had found its form—a Wheel of Life that could expand to contain all the dimensions of our sexual experience.

THE FOUR MAJOR PATHS OF THE ISIS WHEEL

The paths of the ISIS Wheel connect all aspects of your sexuality with all aspects of your life—physical, mental, emotional, and spiritual. As you can see from the diagram, these paths interconnect through the Center, which is wide open to them all.

The ISIS paths don't always follow the rigid boundaries shown in the diagram, however. As you travel them in the complex contexts of your own life, they're likely to twist and turn and wend, or detour or bump, or even come to dead ends. Sometimes following them can feel like slogging through a wilderness. Occasionally you get a straight shot to bliss.

As you travel your personal ISIS paths, you may find yourself traveling them one at a time. For instance, some sexual encounters feel totally physical—have you ever wanted to rip your partner's shirt just to get skin contact? Some feel almost entirely emotional—like when you tenderly tiptoe into each other's hearts after a long absence. But sexual experience is complex, and most often your ISIS boundaries merge. Maybe the love you feel for your partner sends your physical pleasure over the top. Or memories of abuse immobilize your body in mid-orgasm. Or your partner's soft whispers melt your soul. Or old good-girl messages filter through and stop your hand from reaching out to touch your partner's genitals. These are all sexual scenarios women have confided to me. And it's possible that you might experience every one of them, or your own version of them, in what seems to be the same moment of time. When that happens, every bit of you is involved, and you feel as if you're traveling all the ISIS paths at once.

Still, the paths of the ISIS Wheel do have defining characteristics. These are outlined below, and in the chapters that follow we'll explore each one in detail. Some of these paths may seem instantly familiar to you—most women recognize the physical and emotional paths of their sexual experience. But some women wonder what the mental or spiritual paths may have to do with sex. If this is true for you, please don't think there's something wrong with you. The point of diagramming the ISIS Wheel is to make all of the paths equally visible, whether or not they seem to be primary to your sexual experience right now.

The physical path: A full range of sensory experience—smell, taste, touch, sight, and hearing. Movement and stillness. Comfort and safety. Arousal, orgasm, and other physical pleasures. The physical ISIS experience is characterized by heightened senses—brighter colors; increased sensitivity to touch, taste, smell, and hearing; exquisite awareness of how all parts of your body connect.

The ISIS Wheel of Sexual Experience

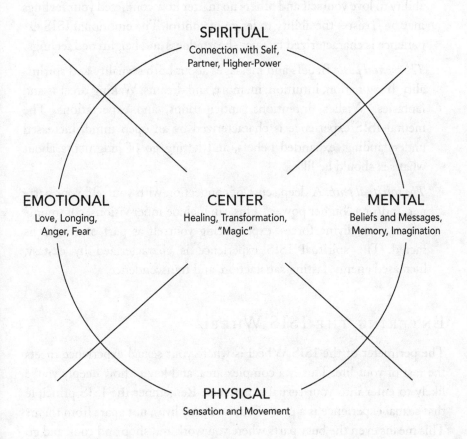

SPIRITUAL
Connection with Self,
Partner, Higher-Power

EMOTIONAL
Love, Longing,
Anger, Fear

CENTER
Healing, Transformation,
"Magic"

MENTAL
Beliefs and Messages,
Memory, Imagination

PHYSICAL
Sensation and Movement

The emotional path: A full range of feelings—love, passion, longing, anger, and fear. Whatever touches your heart. Empathy—the ability to feel what others feel. Compassion—the Dalai Lama describes this as the ability to love yourself and others no matter how conflicted your feelings may be. Trust—the ability to let go of control. The emotional ISIS experience is characterized by open-heartedness and heightened feelings.

The mental path: Beliefs and messages about both sexuality and spirituality. Imagination, intuition, memory, and dreams. Waking dreams and fantasies. Wishes, intentions, anticipations, and expectations. The mental ISIS experience is characterized by an open mind, increased understanding, expanded beliefs, and letting go of judgments about what sex should be like.

The spiritual path: A deep sense of connection with yourself, your partner, and/or a "higher power." This can include inner visions, communication with divine forces, experiencing yourself as part of all that is sacred. The spiritual ISIS experience is characterized by ecstasy, increased energy, lasting satisfaction, and transcendence.

ENTERING THE ISIS WHEEL

The perimeter of the ISIS Wheel is where your sexual experience meets the rest of your life. This is a complex area, and key to how deeply you're likely to enter into your sexual experience. Remember the ISIS principle that sexual experience is a part of our everyday lives, not apart from them? This means even the busy parts where you work and shop and cook and go to school and worship and care for young children and elderly parents and sick friends—and on and on—all of which involve our bodies, minds, hearts, and spirits.

There are times when life feels unutterably good. The sun is shining, the birds are singing, you're ready to open up and let go into sexual pleasure. But sometimes life seems to grab you by the throat. You're not so likely to open up to sex if you're racked with worry over whether or not you can pay the rent or feed your kids tomorrow. Suppose your teenager is on drugs and you keep expecting a phone call from the police—or the hospital?

The physiological models of sexual response don't factor in these crucial questions of sexual context, let alone any conflicting messages we may bring from childhood into our present sexual encounters. Most sex therapists do factor them in, however. For some years I've belonged to an innovative group of psychologists and sociologists who have written an insightful book about how our social contexts affect our sexuality. The essays in *A New View of Women's Sexual Problems* discuss sex in terms of our health, safety, economics, race, sexual orientation, and other life issues we bring to our experiences on the ISIS Wheel.

Given that you are open to exploring your sexuality at this time in your life, let's prepare to enter into the ISIS Wheel. Here's where you begin to focus not only on specific activities but on how sex feels and what it means to your body, your relationships, and every other aspect of your life. Here, at the edge, you can be a little tentative, not fully committed to jumping in. Some women feel safer at the edge because they can jump out faster.

The ISIS Wheel reflects the reality that not all sexual experiences are equally deep. Much of what we call "sex" remains near the perimeter, where you can cruise along well under the speed limit. Here you can begin to sense your own rhythms. You may flirt, make eye contact, relax some tensions of the day. You may feel physically aroused. You may breathe somewhat heavily. Here, near the edge, you may even feel the spasms of orgasm. Maybe not the kind that rock your soul, but compelling enough to remind you that you have a body and that it feels wonderful to let go.

You can hang out indefinitely at the perimeter of any one of the ISIS paths. But when you're ready to explore sex more fully, there are several ways of beginning your journey to the Center. You might begin soulfully. An ISIS woman from Pasadena, California, writes that she enters the deeper levels of sex through looking meltingly into her lover's eyes. Or you can seek a safe emotional passage. Like so many ISIS women, you may need to be well listened to, and also to know that you're the only one on your partner's mind. Or physical contact may be what leads you in, as is true for many women— when physical contact is caring. I love the comment of the ISIS woman who says, "I can read touch and know what it means."

You may find you need some kind of support to begin your ISIS journey. In the best of all possible worlds you'll get this kind of support from your partner, if you have a partner. But support can come from other sources, too. Women's groups have encouraged generations of us to define ourselves sexually—especially around knowing what it is we want and don't want. You can find specific sexual enrichment groups by using the resource section of this book. While these kinds of groups may not be for everyone, they may be just the ticket for some of you. Finally, cleaning out your body and cleaning up your act is a prime way to prepare for your journey to the Center. Numerous ISIS women speak of the importance of recovery from problems with alcohol, drugs, caffeine, sugar, and other substances that clog the body and cloud the judgment.

As you become more and more engaged in your journey, you'll enter more deeply into the ISIS Wheel. Here you feel pleasure flood your body. Your heart melts. The outside world recedes. Clock time speeds up and slows down as if the sorcerer's apprentice were at the controls. You've entered the land where deep and comprehensive orgasm dwells, the kind that can produce hours of delightful aftershocks and a lifetime of memories. Then again, orgasm may be just a way station for you, not the be-all and end-all. You may begin to see your sexual goals in a whole new way— well beyond physical orgasm and into the realm of heart and soul. A colleague I interviewed for *Women Who Love Sex* had a high-hearted way of summing up this urge for something beyond orgasm: "To hell with happiness, I want ecstasy!"

As you move toward the Center, sexual energy moves beyond what we usually think of as the limits of "sex." It can become a potent force for awakening and healing. "Sometimes sex has been the most intense after sorrow," writes a seventy-two-year-old counselor from Santa Monica, California. She goes on to say, "Being in union in love becomes spiritual instantly." And she recites a litany of what this means to her: "Love returned, given, shared, expressed, being understood, cared for, challenged, taught."

Her comments move me because they connect with so many other stories women have shared with me about how sexual relationship helps heal bottomless grief. They also connect me with my own life experience, where I've found that depths of grief and despair can ultimately intensify the joy of letting go into pleasure—not only by way of contrast, but because they open up deeper avenues of feeling and understanding. I'm not the first person ever to understand that grief and pleasure are made from the same cloth. This is one of the great paradoxical truths. The poet William Blake eloquently expresses it in his prophetic "Auguries of Innocence": "Joy & Woe are woven fine / A Clothing for the Soul divine."

IN THE CENTER

As you near the very center of the ISIS Wheel, you enter a kind of high-definition Oz where everything seems vibrantly colored. "A place neither of us has ever seen before," writes a forty-four-year-old massage therapist from Scottsdale, Arizona. You may find, as she does, that it's also a place of mystery and paradox where opposites merge in an uncanny way: "We feel as if we leave our bodies in mind and spirit but feel intense physical pleasure and ecstasy."

Like all levels of the ISIS Wheel, the experience of the Center differs from person to person and time to time. It's yours to define. You may experience opposites, like the woman above. You may feel a sense of oneness and integration, shapeshifting, and timelessness. You may experience extraordinary light—and lightness of being. You may find yourself communing profoundly with your partner, and with yourself. A forty-one-year-old survivor of sexual abuse describes it this way:

An inner explosion of energy . . . culminating in a sort of white-light explosion in my head, that was sublime. . . .What "it" is, I don't know. But it leaves me feeling a sort of awe mixed with tenderness for all of humanity. Like I get it all—why we're here—why I'm here. It all makes sense. I see my purpose. I feel it. I know it. I "grok" it. And I am deeply satisfied, content and renewed. Loved. In Love.

Each journey to the Center can encompass your whole life. There's no past and no future here, only a greatly expanded now. One woman calls her journey to the Center a "divine right." Truly there is divinity here. I've often thought it's no wonder so many of us cry out "Oh God!" at the moment of sexual ecstasy. It's a place of clarity and vision, of vastness, of unconditional love. A forty-nine-year-old secretary from Roanoke, Virginia, writes, "The spiritual/sexual ecstasy is so overwhelming, tears flow from my eyes." She describes the Center as a place where she finds a degree of peace beyond her understanding: "Chaos is everywhere *else*."

Discovering the core of our sexual energy can open up a sudden conversation with God—or whomever or whatever we consider to be a primary source of goodness, power, and grace. I included a question about this in the ISIS survey: "Have you ever experienced God at a moment of sexual ecstasy?" Almost half of all the women who responded to the survey said yes. Hundreds of these women then wrote letters describing encounters with powers and energies beyond themselves. Their stories appear throughout the book, and especially in chapters 8 and 9. If you want to explore these kinds of mystical experiences from another point of view, I recommend Jenny Wade's book, *Transcendent Sex*. She offers both a personal and a scholarly take on what happens when lovemaking opens the veil between the everyday world and the wondrous worlds beyond.

This merging of sexual wholeness and divine grace makes a profound statement about the transformative power of the Center, of the meeting of body, mind, heart, and soul. At a sexology conference recently I spent a lively evening with colleagues speculating about how our world might be different if our international leaders truly understood these complex connections—how our intimate relationships really do serve as a basic pattern for all our relationships. Would political relationships resolve themselves in a more trusting way?

We can't answer this global question. But we can perhaps answer this question for our own relationships. How might broadening your attitude toward sex affect your life? You can begin moving toward that knowledge by knowing where it is you're starting from.

BEGIN WHERE YOU ARE

In group settings I ask women to walk around the circle until they locate the ISIS path that reflects the sexual issues that are most present for them—physical, mental, emotional, or spiritual. If you apply this to the circle of your own life, this means taking a deep breath, putting both feet on the ground, straightening your spine, putting this book aside, and focusing on what's happening for you right now.

Maybe you're in an exciting new relationship and overwhelmed by emotions you've never felt before. Maybe you'd like more affection and empathy, or freedom to make noise, or the courage to say yes to something you've always said no to before. Maybe you long to conceive a baby or be nurtured and babied yourself. Maybe you don't have a partner and are looking—or maybe you've decided your favorite partner is yourself. Perhaps there are problems you feel you need to explore further—anger with your mate, or that old bugaboo "sexual dysfunction." (We'll have more to say about that in chapter 9.) For some people the past is what is most present for them. If this is true for you, you might choose to explore unresolved issues from long ago.

Whatever path you choose, it's only a beginning. You don't have to stay there and you certainly don't have to feel trapped there. We'll find out in the next chapters how the path on which you start your sexual journey can connect you with all the other paths of the ISIS Wheel.

CHAPTER FIVE

SKIN HUNGER AND OTHER SENSUAL APPETITES

Your Physical Journey

MOST OF US BEGIN our sexual journey on the physical path. We're conditioned to think of sex in physical terms—intercourse, arousal, orgasm, heavy breathing, genital stimulation—sensation, sensation, sensation. But ISIS women say their physical responses can range far beyond these sensations to reach a magical tipping point where the physical becomes emotional, spiritual, and universal. The ISIS experience doesn't meant that sex isn't physical. It means the physical path is connected with all the others.

THE BODY SPEAKS

If you listen closely to your body, you know it's more than just a sensory receptor that tells you when you need to eat, pee, and pull on a heavier sweater. It's a sophisticated communication center that connects your physical systems to your emotions, insights, and intuition. It's also a teacher, connecting you with the environment that surrounds you. This is the "intelligence of the body," say holistic physicians such as Christiane Northrup, Deepak Chopra, and Andrew Weil.

Tuning into the wisdom of the body is an important part of making the ISIS connection, for our bodies have a variety of ways of communicating our deepest truths. Simply stated, when you feel good about yourself, your body tends to be healthy, open, and flowing, and so do your thoughts and emotions. You feel a sense of balance, energy, and resilience. You're also open to your environment. (I used to wonder why I am so drawn to the ocean. Now I know it's because the ocean's rhythm and flow help my internal rhythms feel flowing and coherent.)

On the other hand, when you feel guilty, ashamed, or disconnected from your life, your body reflects these feelings, and has some striking ways of letting you know about them. Your body can actually *become* those feelings. I've seen this happen in women who have been abused, abandoned, and otherwise hurt. They may be smiling on the outside, but inside they can be in chaos—with depression, ulcers, and arthritis, not to mention sexual problems and difficulty choosing a caring partner. One client said that her body symptoms were so desperately out of her control that she sometimes felt like a schoolteacher in a room full of acting-out teenagers.

Even without the stresses of trauma, you may be holding on to feelings that keep you from fully expressing your sexuality. Have you ever felt fury with your partner and been unable to express it directly? Negative feelings have to go somewhere or they collect in your body, especially in the areas that want to hit and kick and yell. If you hold on to your feelings long enough—and some of us do this all our lives—you can develop physical symptoms, such as a frozen shoulder or sciatica, or find your dentist scolding you for grinding your teeth to nubs. By the same token, uncried tears can turn into sinus problems. Unrequited longing can create heart problems—yes, you really can die from a broken heart.

It may not be everybody's understanding that emotions cause these medical conditions. But the power of the mind both to distress the body and heal the body has been well documented in alternative medicine. In

The Wisdom of Menopause, Christiane Northrup spells out how the auto-nomic nervous system sends thoughts and emotions into cells, organs, and bones, where they literally incorporate, becoming part of the functioning and structure of the physical body.

So any stored feelings can morph into physical symptoms—and can contribute to sexual problems, from low desire to inhibited arousal and orgasm. The point is, if you want your sexual experience to flow and nour-ish you, you can't be saying both yes and no at the same moment in time—reaching out and pulling back, holding on and letting go.

But sexual "flow" isn't always an option for women. In response to neg-ative sexual circumstances of our lives, some of us find that our bodies have gone numb. "Numb and numb-er"—this phrase came to me recently while in a dentist's chair having a root canal, and it well describes how some women say they experience sex. The truth is, many of us walk around with a great deal of emotional pain, and rather than feeling all the hurt, we close ourselves off from it. But this strategy doesn't serve us over the long run. When you close yourself to your pain, you close yourself to all your feelings. Living becomes a matter of grin and bear it. You numb your capacity to feel joy as well. Sex, dental surgery—it all becomes an out-of-body experience.

If any of this describes you, a primary step on your physical path may be to ferret out where those troublesome feelings are lurking in your body, honor them, and let them go. Not a simple task, I know. I can remember sitting in another painful chair many years ago—in the office of my first psychotherapist—smiling and nodding like a Stepford wife and thinking, "If I ever let out all this rage, it'll blow the entire city off the map." I did let it out eventually and it didn't destroy the city of Boston. Over time I discovered many safe ways to discharge rage, from talking with friends, to beating on pillows, to taking it into sacred ceremony where I could offer it to the fire or bury it in the earth, using age-old rites of recycling what is no longer needed. The chapter on ceremony offers suggestions on how you can create similar clearing rituals for yourself.

HEALING YOUR SEXUAL BODY
Opening to ISIS

The good news is that when you can allow yourself to fully experience all your feelings and bring them into your body, you can begin to change the negative imprints of your past, or at least loosen their grip on you. Remarkable incidents of emotional and even physical healing are possible. An ISIS woman describes just such a healing. A forty-three-year-old photographer from Des Moines writes that her chronic heart condition completely disappeared after she connected sex and spirit for the first time. Think about the imagery here. Quite literally, she had a change of heart when she moved from the coldness of her former husband to the warm attentions of her high school sweetheart. What occurred was a full ISIS experience that began on the physical path. (And, by the way, notice that intercourse wasn't the issue for her, certainly it wasn't the goal.)

He talked to me all night long, relaxing me, holding me, looking into my eyes. He said we didn't need to have sex [i.e., intercourse]. There was something better. He taught me . . . I don't know what to call it. I felt completely safe, floating, saw lights, felt the spirituality.

It took her ten years to speak about this transformative encounter. "I never heard anyone talk about it [the sex-spirit connection] and was afraid people would think I was crazy." She wrote that she felt "crazy" even during her experience, although paradoxically she said she also felt "completely safe." Only when she opened *New Age* magazine and read the ISIS questionnaire did she feel permission to reveal the details of her adventure into body intelligence. She went on, "It felt incredibly great, but scary. My heart problem just went away, the EKG was totally different. The doctors didn't know why. I did, but couldn't tell them. I was too embarrassed to tell anyone."

Another aspect of body intelligence is how closely ISIS women connect their physical senses with other dimensions of sexual experience—emotional, spiritual, and transformational. Tender touch may literally translate into love and commitment as well as physical pleasure. A twenty-two-year-old researcher from Hagerstown, Maryland, elaborates, "He anointed my skin with light traces of his fingertips. I felt emotionally and physically safe. I felt respected and wanted, and I felt really, truly special."

More good news is that it's possible to nurture body intelligence by creating an atmosphere where it can flourish. "There is divinity in the contact of human touch," writes a forty-three-year-old homemaker from Syracuse, New York. Understanding this transformational power of touching, she was moved to make conscious preparations to give and receive it. She says that she and her husband set aside protected times for weekly lovemaking, then set the scene with music, candles, meditation, and declaring their loving intentions.

A twenty-three-year-old paralegal from New Britain, Connecticut, uses the language of several senses to describe her first experience with a woman lover—"the soft, sweet-smelling skin. The tickling of long soft hair." What puts her experience on the ISIS map is that she says these physical sensations are also "saturated with soul." Her description evokes the majesty of religious ritual: "Long glances into her beautiful face were ecclesiastical." Yet her routes to arriving at these connections are grounded in physical reality. She says deep conversation and friendship helped her build enough trust in the relationship for her to risk connecting body and soul. She also stresses the importance of self-knowledge: "It is my strong belief that people need to travel deep within themselves to find that place where their sexuality lies."

THE ISIS PATH TO ORGASM

There's a tacit agreement in sex research that women have problems coming to orgasm. In the pre-Kinsey days, before we knew how to say "clitoris," the number of anorgasmic women was estimated at a whopping 80 percent. This percentage is steadily dropping thanks to the women's health movement, consciousness-raising books like *Our Bodies, Ourselves*, and maybe even media blockbusters like *Sex and the City*.

But still women seek therapy for problems related to orgasm. Much has been written about how to help us become more dependably orgasmic, and this is not the place to go into those details—you can find them in the excellent books I mention a bit further on. In my experience, our orgasms involve more than hormone levels or smart techniques. They also involve your frame of reference—how you think about sex, how you feel about your body, your personal power, and your partner. Your ability to orgasm may depend on what you call orgasm. Or what orgasm means in your life. Or what you're holding on to that prevents your letting go into orgasmic release.

Our physical orgasms have been documented in earliest infancy, in old age, and everywhere in between. From my clinical perch, I've heard women report orgasm from every kind of stimulation—genital, extragenital, and hanging from the chandeliers. Literally. One of the first couples who ever came to me for therapy reported a wildly energetic sexual lifestyle with one great lack: they both agreed that *she* had never come to orgasm. On taking their sex history I discovered that she was having orgasms on masturbation, clitoral stimulation, oral sex, and yes, once, while he softly stroked her as she dangled herself from a rafter over their bed in their Vermont cabin (okay, it wasn't a chandelier). The only way she wasn't having orgasms was on penis-vagina intercourse. This was a problem for them—because it was the only way they thought *real* orgasms could occur.

The idea that all women are supposed to have vaginal orgasms is a throwback to the early part of the twentieth century, when Sigmund Freud famously published his theories of sexual function. At that time it was assumed that women's sexual pleasure depended primarily on their husbands' pleasure. This meant that women had to orgasm during the act of intercourse or not at all. Freud pronounced that orgasms through clitoral stimulation were a sign of sexual "immaturity." Fortunately sexual science has moved on from this limited notion. For many years now we've understood that some women experience orgasm during the vaginal stimulation that accompanies intercourse, but many women do not. Some women need intense clitoral stimulation, and some are most responsive when they're touched and fondled all over their bodies. For still other routes to women's orgasms, keep reading. Much more will be revealed as this book progresses.

Happily for my highly adventurous couple, we could agree that their problem was an information glitch, not a full-blown sexual dysfunction—

where they might have been convinced she needed behavioral therapy to focus her orgasms on intercourse, or perhaps even hormone replacement to engorge her vaginal blood supply in hopes of increasing her sensitivity to penile thrusting. Once this couple had just a bit of updated information, they walked away holding hands and never came back to my office. A few days later they wrote me an ecstatic thank-you note. This was perhaps my easiest "cure." And one that highlights the importance of education. We're all vulnerable to misinformation about sex because so many messages in the culture tell us that intercourse is the only real way to experience sex and orgasm. Anything else is called "foreplay"—that is, only a preamble to the main event.

So one of your first steps on the physical path may be to research the kinds of information that are relevant for you. The books and websites in the back of this book are a good place to start. The sex-therapy literature is full of excellent guidelines for physical stimulation—from vibrators to nonallergenic lubrication, and from water play and bubblebaths to the storied whipped-cream massage. You can find the latest news on medical conditions, hormones, and pharmaceutical enhancements that might affect your progress on the physical path. You can follow the argument for vaginal orgasm in the newly updated edition of *The G Spot* by Beverly Whipple and others, and the argument for clitoral orgasm in Rebecca Chalker's *The Clitoral Truth*. I routinely send women to *Sex Matters for Women,* a comprehensive woman-friendly guide by sex therapists Sallie Foley, Sally Kope, and Dennis Sugrue. Most recently I'm also recommending Annie Sprinkle's *Spectacular Sex* and Patti Britton's *Art of Sex Coaching* because they're written with a contagious sense of adventure and spiritual exploration along with sound clinical advice. I can also reccommend my book, *Women Who Love Sex,* whose women have some extraordinarily wise things to say about the relationship of emotions and orgasm.

What about ISIS orgasms? These may well begin on your physical path but ultimately they radiate out to encompass all of you—body, mind, heart, and soul. ISIS women talk about "heart orgasms" and orgasms of the mind and spirit. The kinds of stimulation that lead to these all-encompassing orgasmic releases are complex and highly individual.

You may not be able to count on self-help books or even your partner to spell out all that's involved in your orgasms. But you can find a great deal out for yourself. Make some private time and space to get to know your orgasmic self. Where do you begin? How far do you go? How far do you want to go? What *are* your physical limits? The practices that follow may help you understand how starting out on the physical path can lead to an ISIS connection into your orgasms.

Your Extragenital Matrix
Expanding Your Erogenous Zones

Early on in my sex therapy practice I took notes as women talked about exactly where they liked to be touched for sexual arousal and satisfaction. I quickly realized they were talking about much more than the traditional "homing sites"—clitoris, vagina, and maybe breasts. Also at that time I was conducting couples weekends and massage trainings, and noticed that several women in these groups were coming quietly to orgasm when their heads or feet were being stroked or simply held in loving attention. So in 1981, when it came time for my Ph.D. dissertation, I decided to explore how women perceived touch during their peak sexual experiences. Sex-therapy pioneers Masters and Johnson had already coined the term "sensate focus," a systematic method for helping couples identify their repsonse to different kinds of sexual touch. But I wanted much more information. And I wanted to hear it directly from women.

I interviewed fifty women who described themselves as "easily orgasmic"—I felt they'd have plenty of information to offer about positive sexual response. I asked each one to remember intricate details of at least two peak sexual experiences they'd had, one with a partner and one on self-stimulation. Where were they touched during these experiences? What kinds of touch were involved? How did they feel? What was most exciting? What was most meaningful? As I suspected, these women mentioned their vulvas—clitoris and vagina. But they also said their most memorable touch ranged far beyond their genitals. They talked about their fingers, toes, knees, elbows, earlobes, bellies, the small of their backs, the nape of their necks, and on and on and on. And the kind of touch that excited them was not only stroking with the hand. It included nuzzling, nibbling, even tickling with the hair and caressing with the breath. Most interestingly, they talked about the meanings behind extragenital touch—the loving intention, the freedom they felt, the comfort, the sense of oneness with themselves and their partners, the release into orgasm, and beyond orgasm to ecstasy. In short, they were describing what I now understand to be ISIS experiences.

I'm not really a voyeur at heart, but these hundreds of hours of interviews moved me to keep on asking even more questions of women. Eventually they provided the impetus for me to conduct the ISIS survey.

From all of this early observation I developed the Extragenital Matrix—a chart that lists different kinds of touch and pairs them with different areas of our bodies. It's included in the back of this book to give you an idea of the varieties and combinations of touch that might await you on your ISIS path. I invite you to think of these as a set of possibilities, not as achievements to notch on your headboard. Some of these kinds of touch may surprise you. Or you may be familiar with all of them already. In any case, you can double your pleasure by introducing them to your partner, if you have one. The Matrix has been published in several books and has been adapted by Planned Parenthood to help young people get creative about sexual activities that don't include intercourse. It's also been presented widely by sex educator Beverly Whipple, the principal researcher of the Grafenberg spot, popularly known as the G spot—the area inside the vagina that brings extraordinary pleasure to some women. She writes, "People around the world can really relate to the Extragenital Matrix. It makes it much easier for them to realize what I mean when I talk about sensuality and sexuality being so much more than the genitals."

ADVENTURES WITH YOUR VULVA

The Kegel Trip

Your genitals are of prime importance on your physical path, too. Kegel exercises (named for Los Angeles gynecologist Arnold Kegel) are a consciousness-raising activity you can do for this wonderful part of your body.

To do "Kegels," you repeatedly tighten and relax your pubococcygeus muscle, or "P-C" muscle, which is located at the base of your pelvic floor. To tighten it, you clench the muscle as if you're trying to stop yourself from urinating. To relax it, you simply let it go. Sex therapists love to recommend Kegels because they're so good for you and they feel good too—a Google search will introduce you to several different techniques. Kegels increase the muscle tone in your vagina and strengthen your pelvic-floor muscles, which support your bladder, uterus, and rectum. All this toning has the potential to make your physical orgasms deeper, stronger, and more satisfying.

Above all (in my experience), Kegeling can act like a kind of "vagina monologue" to increase your relationship with the part of you that's usually kept under wraps, hidden and silent. You may feel intensely sexy. Other intense feelings may also rise to the surface as you connect with your vulva—such as love, connection, fear, longing, or anger. And it's exactly these kinds of feelings that distinguish ISIS orgasms from "performance" orgasms—that is, physical spasms that may be disconnected from the rest of you.

Your Kegels don't have to be mindless, like a treadmill session at your gym. They can become an ISIS experience if you breathe with them and use a little imagination.

Try doing a few ISIS Kegels right now. Take your time. Imagine that you're an exotically hued and tentacled sea creature—and as you breathe in, see if you can suck the sparkling blue-green ocean with all its nutrients into your vaginal opening and all the way up to your heart.

Now breathe out and release your P-C muscle with an enthusiastic whoosh, allowing the ocean to flow back to the source. This may not be exactly the image that moves you, but I trust you get the idea. This is not about mechanistic marching orders—grit-your-teeth, clench-relax, one-two, hut-hut. It's about flow, movement, sensuality, and power. It's about connecting yourself with your body and letting your body connect with the universe around you. Kegeling can be an initiation into the physical path of your ISIS Wheel, and it may lead you in directions that are surprising and delightful.

If you practice Kegel exercises like this—up to 150 each day some doctors recommend—you'll be making a strong bid for sexual health and overall health. No need to schedule special time. Do them on the bus. Do them washing dishes. Be inventive. No one will ever know. Try Kegels when you're paying bills. I sometimes do. It instantly transforms this dreary activity into a secret pleasure. I invite you to practice as you continue to read this chapter.

OUR BELLIES, OURSELVES

At a women's sexuality-spirituality weekend I conducted at Rowe Conference Center in the Berkshires, ceremonial artist Katja Esser, who was assisting with the workshop, surprised us with something new and playful, and profoundly connecting. She'd brought along finger paints and showed us how to create spirals and labyrinths on each other's bellies. Both labyrinths and spirals are ancient symbols of women's power—often seen as paths to the womb of the Great Mother, the center of generativeness, creativity, and erotic pleasure.

In this simple act of body play we were suddenly returning to our roots in an age-old rite of adornment. We laughed and told stories and unloaded years of shame and embarrassment about this core part of ourselves—too fat, too skinny, too flabby, too bloated, too you-name-it. We compared our stretch marks and Caesarean scars. One of us with training in belly dancing showed us how to make our belly labyrinths gyrate and jump. We were in a safe enough place to accept our differences instead of feeling competitive. And miracle of miracles, as we dipped our fingers into the paint pots and decorated one another, most of us found we were touching each other quite intimately—but without any sense of being judged or invaded or otherwise weirded out. Some of us expressed old shame or fear. Some of us felt deliciously turned on. It was the turn-on of self-acceptance and the amazement of sharing such a deep level of our secret selves.

This activity occurred quite spontaneously on a sunny afternoon by a sparkling stream where it was private enough for us to run around like wood nymphs. But indoors in winter works fine too—you can clean up in the shower. Most importantly, you can try this at home if this kind of adventure intrigues you. Try it alone or with your partner—or ask some good buddies over for the afternoon. It may seem like a sidetrack on your ISIS path, but it can touch you to the core. Finger paints, and even body paints, are available at any children's store, maybe even your local five and ten.

SEX WITHOUT SEX
When Orgasm Isn't Your Goal

When sex isn't goal-oriented, the sky can be the limit. (In fact, "skydancing" is the term for ecstatic pleasure in Tantra, an ancient spiritual practice for heightening sexual awareness. We'll say more about Tantra in chapter 15.) Besides, there may be times in your life when genital-orgasmic sex is out of the question—when you have a yeast infection, or don't have a partner, or when you're opting for celibacy. And times when spirituality, or career, or working two jobs to pay the mortgage is more important than physical sex. Even so, our bodies cry out for pleasure. Just look at the sensual treating women do—sunbathing, walking, dancing, watching the slow evolution of a sunrise or sunset. We luxuriate in the sauna, steam, and Jacuzzi at the gym. In summer weather the lure of water is especially strong—bathing, swimming, floating, even watering the garden.

Many women pamper themselves with massages, facials, manicures, and pedicures—one woman admits she can feel the foot treatments go right up to her pelvis. I love being fussed over by my hairdresser—Brigida Guarina is an earth mother who touches my heart as well as my hair. All this pampering is allegedly for beauty, but it also just plain feels good. It provides the caring, nondemanding physical touch many of us lack in our everyday lives.

And there's the erotic power of sensuous foods—preparing them, eating them, feeding your lover and being fed. An exercise I sometimes suggest to clients combines the lustiness of the lobster-eating seduction scene in the movie *Tom Jones* and the soulfulness of a Tantric feeding ritual taught to me by Kenneth Ray Stubbs, whose books explore all manner of sensual pleasures. In its simplest form, you prepare a platter of your partner's favorite fruits, in bite-sized slices suitable for sucking tantalizingly in. You can add a dipping bowl of whipped cream or yogurt. Feed each other fully dressed at your table or naked in your bed—or in your shower, to simplify cleanup.

Some people find blindfolding the partner who's being fed adds a frisson of suspense. For a further touch of kinkiness you can transform your lover into a delectable sundae by laying the fruits decoratively on arms, legs, and belly, then slowly nibbling them one by one. You can play with connecting this exercise with spirit by chanting the "universal sound" of the passionate Foodie—not "Ommmmmmm," but "Yummmmmmmm."

ISIS women report a spectrum of feelings from feeding and being fed. Being the feeder can lend a sense of playful control—of being the "top" in the relationship. Being fed brings some women back to the comforting dependencies—or the devastating neglect—of earliest childhood. Although this exercise is physical, strong emotions may emerge. It's important to honor these emotions as an essential part of nourishing each other.

Even without intercourse or orgasm, the physical path can lead to an oceanic sense of pleasure. A Massachusetts physician in her thirties described an "awesome" experience, in which there was neither intercourse nor genital stimulation. She said this was a conscious choice, to allow for a more open-ended outcome than physical orgasm and to let body intelligence lead her where she needed to go. Nakedness, massage, and sensual exploration morphed into "skydancing."

[We focused on] intense connection through eye-gazing and deep soulful kissing, profound "synesthetic" experiences of sitting in each other's laps and finding all of our senses cross-wired, feeling "synergy"—the presence of more than us in the space [as if we were] channeling spirit.

Her example may be out of the ordinary, but it holds value even for women who don't—or can't—commit their lives to exploring the far reaches of sex and spirit. The great lesson of the physical path is that your body is a trove of emotional and spiritual treasures, great and small. Your body is a great connector. It doesn't stop at the skin. For this idea I thank Emilie Conrad, the founder of Continuum, an innovative approach to experiencing the fluidity of our bodies. Whether you explore your physical path by yourself or with a partner, you're opening your body to ISIS, to integrating sex with what is most meaningful in your life.

In Praise of the Body *and* the Soul

Several years ago I attended a weekend workshop led by Sobonfu Somé, a spiritual teacher from the Dagara tribe in West Africa. The question arose: What does it mean to be fully embodied? We decided to let our bodies speak the answer. We went around the group giving voice to what we felt about our bodies, and a kind of free-verse poem emerged. We named it "The Full-Flesh Givers," and I paraphrase it here, with permission from the women, for it holds universal truths.

When our bodies spoke, they expressed praise—for our bellies, our strength in time of struggle, our bravery in breaking cycles of violence, for "doing relationship in a loud way." Our bodies longed for truth, self-acceptance, sharing, giving and receiving pleasure. Our bodies saw beauty in everyday life. Our bodies felt grateful rather than regretting. Our bodies delighted in standing on their own feet, in their own shoes, able to move forward. Our bodies reveled in their passion: "I am furious. I want to be a warrior with a peaceful heart. I want to nurture myself properly, develop myself into a woman who is heard." Our bodies pulsed with creativity: "Giving birth to myself—whether we give birth or not, we all become the mothers." Our bodies resonated with complexity and wisdom: "I have been through motherhood, periods of giving, having shed my skin many times. At fifty-two I have found the love of my life. A Full-Fleshed Woman. That's who I am! My spirit feels like it belongs with the elders."

The truth is, our sexual bodies function not only *because* of our thoughts and feelings but *as* our thoughts and feelings. It's a variation on the concept of "You are what you eat." You are what you think and feel. You are your sexual desires. You are your path to fulfillment. Walking your physical path can lead you into yourself and far beyond. For right now, let's walk into the next path of the ISIS Wheel—the path of the emotions.

CHAPTER SIX

PASSIONATE AND COMPASSIONATE HEARTS

Your Emotional Journey

SEXUAL EXPERIENCE IS AS lush with emotion as it is with physical sensation. The power of sexual feeling can burst our inner barriers and batter down our locked emotional doors. We laugh and cry. We whoop with elation. We purr with coziness. We surrender to heartthrob and awe, heartbreak and rage. We fling ourselves shipwrecked on the shores of joy. This is the emotional path of the ISIS Wheel. It's where your heart opens up along with your body. Where anticipation and excitement meet deep-seated longing. Where joy, delight, and surprise hold hands with passion and compassion. It's the path of emotional love in all its complexity. Poets and scientists agree that how we negotiate this path is one of the greatest mystery stories ever told.

ISIS women say their journey on this path defies exact description. Still, they find words: "Tuned in to life." "Erotic, exotic, clear, sharp, powerful, strong, natural, psychic and beautiful." "The most profound tears I have ever cried," writes a thirty-year-old psychotherapist. "I wept, raged, laughed, prayed," writes a fifty-eight-year-old author from Naples, Florida, who relived an episode of childhood abuse while making love under the stars in the Sierra Nevadas. Far from being a downer for her, she says this event turned into one of the most healing times of her life. In the trusting passion of her lover's arms she was able to release old shame that had fragmented and numbed her sexual feelings.

Women the world over parse the distinction between having sex (perfunctory intercourse) and making love (sexual experience that satisfies emotionally as well as physically). It doesn't take a perfect life to make love (or "make soul," as one ISIS woman terms it). Many of us have imperfect histories—abuse, drugs, alcohol, risky sex. Some of us became mothers before we were ready. More of us than would admit are in shaky relationships now. Yet I've seen it over and over. From the seeming chaos of women's lives emerges such exquisite emotional sensitivity that we're able to retain the experience long beyond the physical fact of lovemaking—as if our hearts have been stroked as well. A thirty-nine-year-old writer from Tucson says:

Sometimes, afterwards, I clean up but don't wash, so I can carry the essence of our pleasure with me all day long. I know this sounds like some cliché romance novel, but it's true. When I am at my sexual/spiritual peak, I am feeling a womanly high. I am the most woman I can be.

The heart path isn't always smooth. Most likely it's littered with obstacles—the underbrush of past loves, quagmires of self-doubt, quicksands of disappointment that can suck you in until you disappear. We all bring along personal baggage on this path—lost dreams, emotional fallout from abuse, negative messages, adolescent wildness. But heart means courage. Walking this path involves the courage to trust, to let go of emotional armor, and to meet yourself as well as your partner.

Think about what you've felt during your most meaningful sexual experiences. Most women say they want to feel better, feel safer, feel caring and cared for. What about you? What are the pulls and consequences? What do you need in order to walk your emotional path? Let's begin the journey.

Safety, a Key to Opening
Your Heart

Safe sex means more than only preventing sexually transmitted infections. An estimated one-third of American women are survivors of some kind of sexual abuse. Sexologists and others are quick to point out that this percentage may be suspect because there are such vast degrees of what constitutes sexual abuse. Surely there's a difference between an inappropriate grope or proposition and years of incest or torture. Besides, there's no objective way of measuring the extent of sexual abuse or what kinds of problems it actually causes. The point remains that few women look to fear, pain, and danger as sexual turn-ons. Most of us need to feel safe before we can venture onto the emotional path.

But where do we learn about emotional safety? Not from the books on how to overcome sexual dysfunction or the manuals on gourmet sex. Probably not from our mothers unless we had extraordinary families who actually talked about sex. The truth is, many of us have to protect our most naked and vulnerable selves by shutting down our feelings, numbing out, dissociating, leaving the scene emotionally and psychically. This is how sex becomes an out-of-body experience. You're also out of your heart and out of your mind. These strategies may help you cope in the short run, but there's a long-term backlash. When you shut down fear and anger, you also shut down desire. In my sex therapy practice I've spent countless hours helping women unlearn some of their self-protections so they can feel the fear and anger. Then they have to move through these emotions until they can feel the flow of desire again. When I worked in the field of recovery from addictions, we had a catchy (but true) saying: "You can't heal what you can't feel."

Once you feel safe enough to set out on the emotional path, you're ready to create conditions of emotional safety. Most of the conditions anyway. You may not be able to control an abusive situation other than to leave or call 911. But there are many situations you can control to make sex feel safer. Is it privacy you need? Do the obvious. Turn off the phone, pull the shades, lock the doors, send the kids to Grandma's, feed the insistent cat. Do you need assurance that you're deeply loved and won't be abandoned? Say so up front. If this feels too scary, write your partner a letter and ask for a time when you can talk together about your needs— and those of your partner. If your partner can't give you the assurance or the time, then seek professional help. Perhaps your needs predate this relationship and there's a piece of emotional work you need to do on your own. This doesn't mean you're crazy or some kind of failure. One of the great truths of sexual relationships is that they bring your deepest issues to the surface so that you have the opportunity to see them, feel them, and heal them.

One of your issues may be to discover why you're in a sexual relationship that feels unsafe. Some women tell me they need safety not from their partners but from their own histories—a seductive uncle, a tight-lipped granny, a rageaholic boyfriend. I once created a kind of "exorcism" ritual for a young couple so they could remove the specter of her disapproving mother from their bedroom. The chapter on ceremony will give you some ideas you can adapt for the intrusive spirits in your life.

If you're beset by fears that seem to appear out of nowhere, it may help you to weave a very personal safety net. Intention can be a powerfully effective boundary. You can surround yourself with white light or wrap yourself in a pink blanket of love. A wise healer taught me to call down a pyramid of protection—using the ancient power of sacred geometry to keep harmful spirits at bay.

So to engage fully in your emotional path, it's important to think about what safety means for you. Be clear. Invoke it for yourself. And enlist your partner so that it doesn't become a secret between you. Chapter 17 offers practical suggestions for updating your sexual history, with love.

CAREGIVING AND CARETAKING

Nurturers of the World Unite!

Mostly it feels really good to give. But how did women win the role of primary givers of love, comfort, and joy? Is it because we're so famously capable of multitasking? Or is it because we're so traditionally linked with food preparation? Or because we're empathizers—sometimes preternaturally able to feel what others feel, able to walk the emotional path in our partner's moccasins?

Empathy is an essential attribute. Without it we'd all be spinning in our separate egos, and how would we ever get close enough to make love? The challenge is to walk the emotional path without losing *yourself* along the way. Part of the divine paradox is that true empathy starts with connecting with your own feelings, your ability to say what you want, what pleases and excites you. It also depends on your ability to set boundaries, to say no as well as yes. Otherwise you can slide into codependency, a relationship that's all give and no take. If you're a true codependent, you put everyone else's needs ahead of your own, sometimes to the point where you don't know what you yourself need, or even feel. And that leaves everyone confused. I like how inspirational writer Vernon Howard sums up how codependency feels: It's "like letting the waiter eat your dinner."

Another problematic codependency scenario is when *both* of you let go of your boundaries at the same time. Double the confusion, double the angst. An ISIS woman writes of an intense affair where exactly that occurred. She calls it love, but it was really a kind of madness during which they both became so immersed in each other that they lost contact with themselves.

We spent endless hours together doing nothing but gazing into each other's eyes and trying to remember what the other might have been saying, because the aura around us was so intense with love, wants, and passion.

Ultimately the intensity terrified them both and they broke off the affair. Still, she writes, "When we occasionally see one another, we start to get lost all over again in each other. But we pull back just before fireworks start to pop!"

One of the great teachings of the emotional path is about balancing your ability to receive as well as to give. The truth is that sometimes it's easier to give than to receive. It can put you in a position of power and control—Big Nurse dispenses the goodies and also gets to set the rules. A need to feel in charge is a healthy human need until it gets out of whack, which it sometimes can in our most intimate relationships. My guess is that a need for control is why some women marry unnurturing men—and stay with them forever. Caregiving is not only a woman thing of course. I know many men who are fabulous nurturers. But some men remain clueless all their lives. It's a learned disability, I think. Would clueless men keep being clueless if women expected them to become emotionally wiser?

The way this kind of care-lessness plays out can be unbearably sad. A childhood friend confided to me, years after the fact, that her husband drew a line down the middle of the bed on their honeymoon and told her never to cross it except for sex. The astounding thing is that she complied for more than a decade—until he left her, claiming she was frigid. There's a depth of cold I've encountered in undernurtured clients. A woman I used to see piled on sweaters and scarves and still shivered, even in my warm office, because her chill came from deep inside her.

I can understand because I was there too, back when I didn't know that women had a choice. I mistook attention for love, and physical desire for heart connection. I was attracted to my first husband because we liked the same books and he wasn't a drunk. I married my second because when he drank, at least he was fun. He could do fascinating parlor tricks like write forward and backward with both hands at once. Long after we'd parted I kept a scrap of paper in his writing-and-mirror-writing that said: *Gina when dressed in red and yellow is the sexiest thing I know.* But drunk or sober, he was never fully present for me. He never understood what I meant by hugs. Clearly I wasn't all that present either, and didn't know how to let him know what I needed.

What I needed was understanding, closeness, and tenderness. I needed commitment, a sense of deep, ongoing connective tissue to link my body, mind, heart, and soul. I needed love—"Thi-i-i-i-i-s much"—to make up for childhood neglect. These needs weren't outlandish. What was outlandish was my sense of desperation about them. I thought I'd die if they weren't all met, all the time, especially during sex. Nobody could measure up, of course, so I ended up broken-hearted, like so many women I know. On the emotional path you can see the shards littering the ground. It's like going on an archeological dig. Oops, there's a piece of this relationship sticking up here. And over there, there's a little corner of that lover.

How do you mend a broken heart? First, you locate it. One way to connect with your heart is through the following exercise.

OPENING YOUR HEART WITH
YOUR BREATH

Place your hands over your heart and make the sound "Aaaaah" as you exhale. Use plenty of clear, steady voice—don't whisper and don't yell. As you do this, see if you can start to feel a sense of warmth or energy radiating from your heart into your palms. Then, with each inhalation, send the energy from your hands back into your heart. Literally breathe the energy in, and breathe it out again as you chant "Aaaaah."

This practice can help you connect with your heart. It can also help you feed it energy. You can deepen this exercise if you consciously release grief with each exhalation, and visualize love and gratitude flowing in with each inhalation. When I do this exercise, after a few minutes I can feel the energy of my heart expanding in waves.

When you begin to open your heart in this way, you can consciously remind yourself how connected your heart is with your sexual feelings. On your next exhalation send your breath down into the energy centers below your belt. Send it into your pelvis—your belly and your genitals. When you inhale, send your breath from your pelvis back up into your heart. Let yourself feel the flow between your heart and your genitals—your emotional center and the center of your physical sexuality. Allow the feelings to flow as freely as they can. You're opening the pathways between your heart and your genitals—and this path may have been rerouted, flooded, or temporarily blocked by any number of experiences from your childhood on.

If any images come up for you, breathe into them and give them life. Some women connect with images of deep love. Some feel immensely sad. Or angry. Whatever may be true for you, keep breathing and keep connecting. But—and this is an important "but"—know that you don't have to feed your feelings of terror or images of violence or abuse. If these begin to feel overwhelming, reroute your breath back to gently opening the channel that connects your pelvis and your heart.

You can extend this exercise still further to connect your heart to the larger world around you, to the earth, and to the sacred. Here you're reminding yourself that your sexual energy is connected with nature and with universal energy. To begin this connection, start by fully contacting the ground. You can stand, sit, or lie down, either inside or outdoors in nature. (Whenever possible, I try to do this exercise outside on a favorite rock, since I find rocks are such potent conductors of earth energy).

As you inhale, breathe the energy of the earth up into your heart, and then send it out again through your pelvis, down through your thighs and knees and out your feet. As you deepen these breaths, allow yourself to feel the energy of the earth flowing into your pelvis and your heart. If you encounter any physical tension or emotional static, send these down into the earth. Don't worry that you might be polluting the environment by dumping your emotional garbage. Instead, think of yourself as actually feeding the earth with your deepest feelings. This may be a stretch—but this whole exercise is a stretch, yes? Perhaps it will help you to know that many indigenous belief systems hold that a primary role of Mother Earth is to consume our negative energy and transform it—think of it as a kind of emotional compost principle. There's even a term for this in the Andean Mesa tradition that I practice. It is *hucha miqui.* "Hucha" means density—that includes your emotional garbage. "Miqui" means digestion. In this tradition, it is the unique gift of Pachamama—Mother Earth—to digest our deepest grief and angst and turn it into rich, life-giving compost.

You can open your heart still further by breathing in the pure light of heaven. Let a shaft of illumination enter through the crown of your head. Open to it. Breathe this light down into your heart, and send it back up again. As you continue your cyclic breathing, allow the energies from the heaven and earth to meet in your heart. Feel them spiral throughout your whole body and out into the universe.

Here, you may find yourself activating the kind of heart energy described by shamanic healer and teacher Oscar Miro-Quesada. He calls it the "high heart." This is a place of altruism and compassion. A place beyond fear, blame, resentment, and victimization. When the Dalai Lama spoke after the attacks of 9/11, he spoke exactly from this high-heart place. When he was asked how to deal with violence and aggression, he responded, "We all want to be happy. And remember, the other person, the other nation, wants to be happy too." What sound counsel for our heart-path journeys. By tapping into love and understanding instead of fear and resentment you can rewrite your past and reroute your sexual journey in the present. And always along the heart path you'll find opportunities to offer compassion for yourself. Sobonfu Somé, another wise and gentle healer, teaches this in her powerful workshops on grief. She urges us to welcome our own wounds and worst habits as our teachers, as gateways to the freedom, health, and prosperity we long for.

To complete this breathing exercise, give thanks to your breath—and to all that your breath contacted. Spend some time reflecting on what you learned—write it in your journal, if that's your style. Be aware of how opening your heart can affect your journey on the ISIS Wheel of sexual experience.

THE POWER OF PLEASURE
The Art of Feeling Good

Another teaching of the emotional path is about taking ownership of the P-words, *power* and *pleasure*. Both of these terms are loaded with controversy in today's society. They appear often in the experience of ISIS women. The kinds of pleasure they describe is the joy of connection—with self, partner, nature, and a power greater than themselves. The kind of power they describe is not power *over* but increased energy and good feeling—the kind of power that wants to share.

Four in five ISIS women say they connect sex and spirit through sharing deep feelings. But how can women share feelings they're not supposed to feel and not supposed to talk about? Annie Sprinkle, a sexologist and performance artist, tackles this problem with insight and humor. She's created a workshop called "Sluts and Goddesses" where women spend a whole weekend exploring the range of emotions embedded in these prime archetypes of sexual power and pleasure. She sets the stage for women to act these roles to the hilt, complete with outrageous costumes, props, and makeup. Says Sprinkle, "I had it and they wore it. It was dress-up time, and over the top." This roleplaying concept is supremely simple, and like so many simple concepts it packs enormous emotional punch. It may not be for everyone, but feedback from women who've been there say their feelings opened up, their sex lives became much more adventurous, and they felt filled with new power. Once you've let your inner slut and goddess out of the closet, you're not so likely to capitulate to a controlling partner. Nor do you shiver with emotional cold. For a full description on how to access these sexual-power archetypes in your own life, read her wonderful sex-life makeover: *Dr. Sprinkle's Spectacular Sex.*

Some women discover these archetypes on their own and manifest them in their own ways. I love what a forty-six-year-old massage therapist from Missouri writes—even though she never took Annie Sprinkle's workshop:

I recently told my sister that I had decided to be a goddess. She of course thought I meant it as a joke, but I was completely serious. It is only because I have reached a point where I know I am part of God and that I am worthy of being worshipped (it only takes one man to worship you to make you a goddess, right?). If he is not here now, he is on his way, and I am going to be ready.

Of course not all ISIS women define pleasure through goddess power (or slut power). What's *your* pleasure? British psychologist Robert McBride offers guidelines for finding your personal "bliss point." It's a kind of sensate focus for your emotions—to help you become aware of needs you may have buried over the years while you were busy pleasing others. Ask yourself, What do I want? How much do I want? How good does it feel? Do I feel better than I did yesterday, last week, last year?

This line of questioning can be extremely helpful for raising sexual awareness. But if you find yourself resisting the idea of a single bliss point—or G spot or magic button—you're not alone. Some women don't like the notion of sexual pleasure being reduced to a single point or spot. ISIS women tend to think in oceanic terms, such as "heart connection with my partner" or "a gift of grace from the universe." Appreciating the power of feeling good is an art because it doesn't obey the logical rules of science.

Any degree of pleasure can be an epiphany on your heart path. Or it can turn into a yawning sinkhole. According to what I call "the law of incredibly shrinking women," we're not supposed to define sexual pleasure for ourselves. So how do you cultivate your freedom to enjoy your expanding sexuality without feeling that someday a fiery dragon is going to make you pay? Ultimately this depends on your feelings about *you*.

ACCEPTING YOURSELF AS YOU ARE

Sexual self-acceptance is a big issue for ISIS women—Carol Ellison's intelligent book *Women's Sexualities* details her survey on how generations of women are able to find it for themselves. How do you develop good feelings about your body and yourself when the culture tells you how you're supposed to look, dress, act, think, speak, eat, smell, make love, and reproduce? The problem goes deeper if you have some kind of obvious "difference," such as a mastectomy, or genital surgery, or a disability that affects how you look or move or feel. And suppose your partner draws a line down the sheet or tells you you're too fat, too thin, too blonde, too dark, too much, too little, too—whatever? It can take courage and determination to look beyond all this outside chatter and define yourself from the inside.

I've often suggested that women begin walking the emotional path by spending quality time looking in a full-length mirror—conversing with themselves and paying close attention to what they say back. This is a conversation you can try with your clothes on—and also naked. Lights on and lights off. Before and after bathing. Before and after masturbating or making love. Notice any differences in how your body feels and how you feel about your body.

The first time I ever did this was during a self-awareness workshop during my doctoral training. Not all Ph.D. sexologists are trained in this experiential way, in case you were wondering. Most learn simply by reading books. But you can't learn everything about sexual feelings by reading books, and this kind of intense self-awareness exercise is typical of how we were trained at the Institute for Advanced Study of Human Sexuality, where I got my doctorate. There were maybe twenty of us in the class and the exercise was being videotaped. One by one, we had to approach the ornate standing mirror in the front of the room. Then we had to take our clothes off and talk about our naked bodies.

To talk with your naked image in the mirror is awkward enough when you're alone in your bathroom with the shades drawn. But to do this as part of a group was deeply terrifying for me. I don't know if it was other people's judgments I feared—I suspect what I feared more was voicing my own judgments about myself. Some women in the class danced and flirted their way through this exercise, but when my turn came all I could do was cry— great honking tears. Ultimately it was way beyond fear or shame or anything else I can put a name to. I think a river of the don't-ask-don't-tell of my proper Bostonian upbringing drained away in those tears, along with an ocean of grief for all women in the world who had ever been objectified and humiliated.

A variation on this exercise comes from the consciousness-raising sessions developed in the 1970s in books like *Our Bodies, Ourselves.* Curl up on your comfy bed with a hand mirror and have a good long look at your vulva—your clitoris, your lips, your pubic hair, your vagina—all those hidden unmentionable places. Say "Hi, Sweetie." Or maybe this isn't the phrase that springs to your lips. Eve Ensler's *Vagina Monologues* spells out the gamut of feelings women have about their vulvas—from joy to fear, pain, and rage. So let your greeting take whatever form is right for you. If this exercise feels gross or uncomfortable at first, I encourage you to try it anyway. The rewards are that you'll go on an emotional journey you may never have been on before—and who knows what discoveries it may reveal to you.

After you've greeted your vulva, let her introduce herself to you. (Some of Ensler's women named theirs in *Vagina Monologues.*) Ask your vulva how she feels about being undressed like this. You can ask her what she feels about oral sex. Intercourse. Masturbation. Do you see her smile? Or does she pucker up and withdraw?

Perhaps she'd like to chat with other vulvas in the neighborhood. Maybe you can find a few good women to join you on a Sunday afternoon with their hand mirrors. (If this feels like too much of a stretch for you, let it go). Or there's a remarkable book of vulva photographs you can look at for reference instead. It's called *Femalia,* and it's published by Down There Press. What a great name. And by all means, read (or better, see) *The Vagina Monologues,* the amazing play that's brought the V-word to conversations all over the world. It's often performed around Valentine's Day, especially on college campuses.

Re-envisioning Your Sexual Self-Image

Over the years I've witnessed so many clients in agony over their sexual self-image that I developed a sneaky technique that's helped many of them feel instantly better about themselves. It's based on the Wizard's First Rule, which is that people believe what they want to believe. You know how powerful that simple statement is if you've ever tried to convince someone to vote for the candidate *you* think can run the country best. In this culture, most people believe what they see on television. The person on TV is the authority, the expert, the news anchor, the Dr. Phil who can solve all your relationship problems.

My technique is also based on the theory that if you feel fully connected with your emotions, you're much more apt to feel powerful. This may sound obvious, but it's actually at the foundation of some transformative therapies such as Neurolinguistic Programming (NLP) and Eye Movement Desensitization and Reprocessing (EMDR), which have helped many thousands of people regain a positive self-image.

So here's how you can create your own heart-path sexual-self-image reality show—starring YOU. It's a variation on the mirror exercises. What you need is about an hour of privacy and a video camera you can hook up to a TV monitor. (You can use a traditional video camera or a digital video recorder.) This is an exercise you can try at home by yourself, but it helps to have a trusted partner, friend, or therapist hold the camera for you and gently direct the timing.

Step 1. (Five minutes) Record yourself talking about how you feel you don't measure up as a sexual being. How do you feel ugly, awkward, dysfunctional, unnoticed, unappreciated, uncared for? Let yourself get into it.

Step 2. (Five minutes) Watch the video of yourself complaining. Watch in silence, don't comment just yet. Take in the full essence of that person you see on the screen. What does she look like? How does she sound? Does her body language match what she's saying? Do you believe her? What do you feel as you watch her and hear her story?

Step 3. (Five minutes) Make another video of yourself responding to the first video. This is likely to be the most interesting part. Very often a woman is instantly transformed by seeing herself. I've heard many women respond like this: "That person on the video looks pretty terrific. I had no idea I looked that good. Wow. That's really me, eh? So what am I complaining about?" Using video images in this way can allow you to clean house and update your self-image. It can insert a positive picture in place of the negative one you've been carrying around all these years. If this happens, put your new image in the pocket next to your heart and go home. Mission accomplished.

There's another major way I've heard women respond to watching themselves voice their sexual complaints: "That person is lying." This response seemed extraordinary to me until I fully understood the NLP research on subtle eye movements. It shows that you and only you can look yourself in the eye and discern whether the sad story you've been telling yourself all these years is the truth. Perhaps it's not. Perhaps it's a story you've made up to protect yourself, to fit yourself into the cultural narrative—that women are less sexual than men. On this video you may actually catch yourself in a big fat lie that even you never knew you were telling.

If this is so, it doesn't mean you're a bad person. This kind of truth bending is something women do to give themselves the illusion of belonging, even when we know we don't really belong. But the camera doesn't lie. And the truth may be that you're *not* ugly, dysfunctional, and invisible. You may see that you're really beautiful, juicy, and full of life. So put *that* image in your heart pocket and take it home. And take some time to sit with your feelings. And remember to breathe.

Step 4. (Five minutes) Watch the video of your response to the video of your complaints. This is often enough to complete the learning and update your sexual self-image. If you need to keep going, video another five-minute conversation with your self—and another and another—for as long as you feel it's helpful. The point is, on the issue of your sexual self-image you are your own best therapist and coach. No amount of feedback from others is as deeply convincing as the feedback you can give yourself.

Exploring your sexual self-image is a natural entry to the next path of the ISIS Wheel. So when you're ready, let's move to the mental path—how your physical and emotional journeys connect with the sexual messages you receive from the culture and how you develop your deeply held sexual beliefs.

CHAPTER SEVEN

BELIEFS AND MESSAGES

Your Mental Journey

PHYSICALLY AND EMOTIONALLY charged as sexual experience may be, it's also profoundly influenced by our minds—by our beliefs about how we should express ourselves sexually. And so we enter the mental path of the ISIS Wheel. When the path is clear, our minds can flow with new experiences. We're able to let go of pleasure-killing *should*s and *ought*s. We can be discerning about our sexual choices rather than judgmental about them.

It's common currency (among sex therapists anyway) that sexual desire, excitement, and passion actually begin in our minds. It's often written that the brain is our most important sex organ—it's not all about the call of the genitals. The problem is, we're not always able to use this most important organ to its full capacity. We may find ourselves trapped in limiting belief systems about what it is we're really passionate about. We waffle around in a cultural trance about how sex ought to be. What's okay, what's not okay. What feels good, what doesn't feel good. When, how, why, and with whom sex should and shouldn't be. Our memories and dreams can cloud these issues rather than illuminate them. Our imagination and intuition can bow to the dominant myth—that women don't really deserve that much pleasure. We can fuse sex in the present with sex in our past. For women who carry any kind of sexual wounds, it may seem that sex will always be the way it was—a perpetual treadmill of clueless partners, pain, heartbreak, betrayal, and ominous headnoises. No wonder so many women say, "Not tonight, dear."

I empathize. For many years I wandered around in my own trance. Even after I was married, sex was one of those facts of life that was scary and fascinating, but I knew little about its real meaning, power, or purpose. I was born at the end of the Great Depression in Boston, a city dreary with coal smoke and stiffly starched attitudes. "Banned in Boston" was the catchphrase of the time. The major sexual message was "nice girls don't." In fact, most of us *didn't*, and we didn't talk about it either. In my household there was lots we didn't talk about (such as our venerable family traditions of alcoholism, divorce, and suicide), and we certainly didn't talk about sex.

I learned early that "nice girl" meant ashamed, confused, and absolutely mum about sexual feelings. This message was reinforced by one of my treasured possessions—a brass statue of the See No Evil, Hear No Evil, Speak No Evil monkeys covering their eyes, ears, and mouth with their little paws. I understood beyond doubt that "evil" meant any kind of sexual involvement. I knew all about "Just say no" long before Nancy Reagan popularized the phrase or the Silver Ring Thing became the abstinence-dujour program for American youth. I was living it.

Granted, this was the pre-Kinsey generation—well before the sexual revolution that supposedly shook America out of its sexual dark ages. But I'm hearing lots of the same old songs from women in my practice today: Don't ask for what you want. Don't make noise. Don't ask, don't tell. What will my priest/rabbi/minister say? What will the neighbors say? To complicate matters now, we have a conflicting set of messages to deal with as well—titillating images from television, magazine ads, almost everywhere. You can't escape them in our sexualized postmodern culture. They attack the minute you open your e-mail. The other morning I received yet another ad offering chemical relief for my dry vagina or limp penis. "Click Here to Increase Your Sex Life! For Women—Gives You Great Bone-Jarring, Earth-Moving, Climb the Ceiling, Technicolor Orgasms! For Men—You Will Get a Rock-Hard Pump!" (I am not making this up.)

These messages are always about performance and they almost always objectify women. They tell us: "Look sexy, act sexy, but for God's sake don't actually *be* fully sexual." What's a girl or woman supposed to believe? The messages are screwy. And as a colleague who wishes to remain nameless points out, girls and women are always the first to get screwed.

The power of these double messages came home to me full blast with the publication of my book *Women Who Love Sex*. The title was designed to challenge the notion that women are congenital naysayers and gatekeepers, and to show how deliciously lusty we can be, given the right conditions. Instead, it ended up serving as a Rorschach for readers' attitudes. Some readers loved the notion of women loving sex instead of hating it and said, "Count me in! I'm one of those!" But all too often I heard, "Waddaya mean women-who-love-sex? You mean sluts and bimbos? You mean women who love sex *too much*?" One TV interviewer actually waved the title at the camera and said (wink, wink), "What is this, some kind of *phone book*?"

The point is, the way we think about our sexual experience may be hammered into shape long before we have a chance to develop our own ideas. We can become molded by messages that seep through the cultural airwaves—religion, medicine, and the media. Even sex surveys collude by portraying women as less interested in sex than men—and more dysfunctional. Sometimes these messages are strong enough to twist our thoughts and break our hearts and spirits. They're tough for sex educators and therapists to counter, no matter how earnestly we may try. My colleague Leonore Tiefer does the most interesting job I know of putting the good-girl/bad-girl argument into perspective, and she does it with brilliance and humor. I heard her bring a crowd of students in Orlando, Florida, to a standing O (ovation, that is) by showing Andy Singer's says-it-all cartoon —of "Extra Virgin" and "Cheap Slut" olive oil. It's on the next page— picture it blown up to wall-size in a darkened auditorium.

Just look at the teachable moments in these images: The "Extra Virgin" olive oil possesses everything desirable. It's organic, imported, and cold-pressed. It's tightly corked and worth much more than its counterpart. "Cheap Slut" falls well short of these standards. It's heavily processed— with multiple *hot* pressings—and made in New Jersey with a screw-off cap. It's not quite a dime a dozen, but it's definitely priced to sell. These images highlight the cultural double standards that affect our body image and self-worth and ramp up the voice inside that says, "You're not doing it right."

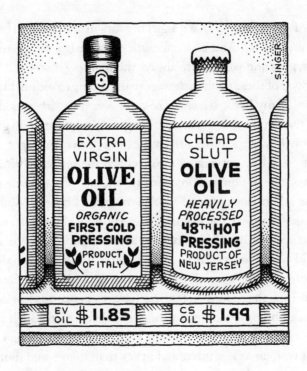

Beyond Stereotypes

Waking Sleeping Beauty

Maybe you reached adulthood knowing you're powerful and worthy, sexually and spiritually whole. Believe it or not, some women do, despite the risks, put-downs, taboos, and misunderstandings. Perhaps you had parents who modeled joy in their physical and spiritual relationship with each other. Maybe your community wasn't bound by stern religious morality or tight-lipped customs. You may have been lucky enough to meet a partner early on in life who delighted in you and in pleasure and helped you feel safe enough to explore your sexuality as a source of connectedness, health, and personal power. There are inspiring stories everywhere if you search them out.

But most of us have to make our way through a jungle of conflicting messages that affect our partners as well as ourselves. This means we sometimes have to be inventive enough and courageous enough—and even desperate enough—to leap into the sexual unknown. For some women this means years of therapy and finding a new mate. For others it means seeking out books, DVDs and videos, and other forms of information. For still others it means turning their back on the religion they grew up in to find a spiritual practice that honors body as well as soul. Some women leap simply because they feel they must. They have no choice but to plumb the depths of their own passion and their own spirituality.

Others allow their bodies to wake them from their sleeping-beauty trance. As I write this sentence from a perch overlooking the Pacific Ocean, I'm suddenly blasted by bone-shaking tunes from a nearby car. Four twenty-somethings hop out smoking cigarettes and start rocking to the beat and the sunset and each other. Perhaps this is what it takes to wake them up, rock them into new patterns.

At the other end of the spectrum are the hundreds of feisty older women in my practice and in the ISIS study who say they've lived long enough to be able to pooh-pooh the messages that kept them tightly laced when they were younger. For these women, menopause and white hair don't represent the end of sex. They're a passport to freedom. I could fill a book with wise and wonderful material from these women (and yes, I'm planning to do that). For now, suffice it to say that my heart goes out to the late-blooming seventy-three-year-old who writes that her day for pleasure has finally come: "Time to wake up and feel the tush!"

And that's what the mental path is about. Waking up, taking charge, opening to new possibilities, letting them take you where you need to go—by yourself or with a partner. Everyone can find her own way. It's a question of activating your sexual imagination so you find the jumping-off point that's right for you.

TAPPING INTO YOUR SEXUAL IMAGINATION

Your sexual imagination includes a continuum of responses. These range from negative memories, fears, flashbacks, nightmares, and premonitions to positive memories, anticipations, wishes, dreams, and fantasies. All of these are crucial to your sexual attitudes. They help you perceive nuances of excitement and pleasure. They help you distinguish pleasure from pain. They lead you to accept your social conditioning, or move beyond it. They help you form erotic relationships and experience the full bloom of ecstatic spiritual union.

Let's look at dreams. A thirty-seven-year-old music therapist writes, "My greatest teachers about sex are my dreams. I ask questions and my dreams answer them." So let's consider your dreams as your teachers. Not only the overtly sexy dreams where you're shacking up with an old lover or rolling around in strawberry fields with your favorite rock star. But the nonsexual ones as well, where you meet friends and mentors, ancestors and animal allies all offering their own brand of sexual wisdom if only you listen and take them to heart.

Dreams are intimately connected with other levels of consciousness—fantasies, daydreams, dreamtimes, and meditations. The lines between them can sometimes blur. A telltale difference is that sexual fantasies are still relatively taboo for women, so you may find yourself shy about expressing them, or admitting them, or even recognizing them for the lusty energy and soul they can impart.

Visualizing new and possibly taboo experiences can be exciting whether or not you act on these experiences, says Wendy Maltz, a wise sex therapist in Eugene, Oregon. Her wonderful book, *Private Thoughts,* goes beyond cliché plots and characters. It's woman-positive and sex-positive and aims to help you build your sexual self-image and sense of play.

One of the ways I've helped clients free themselves from old, limiting messages is to encourage them to enter an imaginary Magic Shop of their own making. You can try doing this right now. This enchanted space is crammed from floor to ceiling with sexual and spiritual images, activities, and devices—a full spectrum, from black leather to feathery angel's wings. Take a moment to fill this Magic Shop with your own ideas and images. Make a list right now in the margin of this book if you like. These items can be racy, or plain vanilla, or quite forbidden. You don't have to tell anybody what they are. You can pick and choose, mix and match. You can take a sparkly wand and transform them to suit your mood—Harry Potter meets sex therapy. It's fun. It's illuminating. And it can free up your conversation about sex—especially the conversation you have with yourself.

In your sexual imagination is a happy paradox. You can enter a world of freedom, and you can also exercise utter control. You can try out new behaviors from dress-up to bondage and discipline. You can shift your sexual orientation or your gender. You can play with any partner you want. Writer and activist Cecilia Tan speaks to this state of affairs in an article she wrote for *Sojourner* in 1999.

> . . . it's mine, because I'm the one who controls it . . . all the things I'd be afraid to ask a real world lover to do, maybe, or all the things my society tells me are naughty or bad or illegal. But hey, if I'm tied up like Penelope Pitstop, in my fantasy, I am guilt-free. My libido gets what it wants, it's the engine that drives the fantasy machine, and I get to feel stronger about my sexual identity because I've accepted that my fantasies are okay.

Sexual imagination is more than just dreams and fantasies, though. It can improve your lovemaking skills and deepen the emotional and spiritual connection with your partner. You can use it as the ultimate in safe sex. Whether you read romance novels or work the Internet, you can indulge in steamy relationships without having to fuss with latex or face a real person in the gray light of morning.

You can also use visualization, meditation, and fantasy to relieve a raft of ills—shame, fear, fatigue, flagging desire. You can reframe or transcend your past wounds by visualizing healthy, loving relationships in the present. In the practice of sex therapy, visualization techniques are a standard treatment for some kinds of vaginal pain and for vaginismus—spasmodic contractions of the vagina that make intercourse impossible. You can even use your sexual imagination to take you to the land of spontaneous orgasm—a rarified realm where you experience orgasm without any physical touch.

Spontaneous orgasm is a secret that has been well kept from the American public. It doesn't fit the performance model, so most sex researchers don't ask about it. But I've asked about it, and countless women have responded, "Yes!" They say it can happen anywhere—in sleeping dreams and in the waking state—in daydreams, meditation, guided imagery, flashes of insight, immersion in nature, reading, watching videos, body-watching, eye contact with a lover, breathing together, conversing, talking on the telephone, or driving a car. It can happen in a paroxysm of Tantric ecstasy, or just walking down the street.

One woman I interviewed for *Women Who Love Sex* gave it a catchy name: "Oh, you mean *thinking off.*" She said she experienced it often and it made her realize what a powerful person she was. "All I have to do is use my imagination, and then SHAZAM! It's something nobody can take away from me. Even if I end up in a Catholic nursing home like my grandmother, I'll have my secret weapon. And they'll never know."

Having interviewed so many women who *can*, and *do*, I considered writing a lighthearted book titled *The Thinking Woman's Guide to Thinking Off.* Instead I took the high road and joined a team of laboratory researchers at Rutgers University in the early 1990s to document that women are able to come to orgasm on imagery alone. The report was published as a peer-reviewed article, so science now acknowledges the existence of spontaneous orgasm. But what is its significance? What occurs in women's lives when their minds connect with their bodies in this way? A journalist once told me a lovely story that led me toward an answer. In the midst of interviewing me about my work she leaned over and confided that she'd once come to orgasm in the palm of her hand.

"The palm of your hand?"

"When I was first falling in love with my husband," she said. "It's one of the reasons I decided to marry him. I thought if I feel *this* good around him, it's got to be a sign."

"Please tell me more," I urged her. One of the perks of being a sex therapist is that you can probe for details without seeming to be entirely prurient.

"We were sitting at one of those long tables in a public library," she said, "and suddenly I felt like patting his cheek. But it happened before I even touched him. I was just reaching toward his face when I felt this bolt of energy shooting out of my right hand."

"How did you know that was an orgasm?"

"It was explosive and warm and it went all through my body and it felt wonderful. But the most amazing part was what happened when the after-shocks wore off. I flashed back to a memory of what sex had been like with the first man I lived with. I wondered why in the world would *he* come to mind? He was mean. He used to force himself on me. Then I was conscious of that pulsing still in my hand—and all at once it was as if my body remembered. I used to go rigid whenever he approached me. That way I wouldn't have to feel anything. I'd stay all clenched up like this." She held up two tightly wrapped fists for me to see.

Then she laughed and shook out her fingers until they relaxed again. "But it's totally different now. My husband is such a gentle guy, there's nothing scary about him at all." she said. "I feel so much better about myself now that I can let myself open up."

This experience had many meanings for this journalist. Clearly it gave her pleasure—enough to influence her decision to marry. It also provided a bolt of insight to help her distinguish between the kind of love that nurtures and the kind that hurts. Her flashback was a beacon that served as a release of past pain and an injunction to stay open to present pleasure.

The image of an open hand runs through many women's accounts of their sexual opening. It's connected with the ability to open up their entire beings—to give and receive is the power of an open hand, not a closed fist. Contrast this image of open-handed power with the pornographic or stock media images of women as sex kittens—"Grrls" with pouty lips, spread legs, and sharpened claws.

The mental path of the ISIS Wheel is more than a route to orgasm, or a cog in Cecilia Tan's "fantasy machine." When you walk it consciously, you enter an inner sanctum of body and soul, a constellation of sexual attitudes, a defining imprint, a fulcrum for erotic transformation. Your sexual images are yours to have and hold, long beyond the excitement of the moment. They lodge deep in the wellspring of your memory.

Mind-body research reminds us that memories inhabit our bones, muscles, and cells, as well as our cognitive faculties. Wilhelm Reich, the founder of bioenergetic therapy, famously labeled these "body memories." Our memories also inhabit the bioelectric energy fields within and around our physical bodies. These are "emotional and spiritual memories," according to physicist Valerie Hunt, who discusses them in *The Infinite Mind*, her foundational work on the vibrations of consciousness. Still further, visionary psychiatrist Carl Jung proposed that we all possess a collective memory, or "collective unconscious," a shared link with our ancestral roots.

In truth, you can come to many of these same conclusions if you spend enough time listening closely to women describe their favorite sexual experiences. Throughout the years of my clinical work I've consistently found that all these levels of memory inform our sexual experience—and they do so whether we're aware of them or not. The ebb and flow of memory is at the core of our sexual beliefs and images, our cavewoman appetites, our infant instincts to nuzzle and suck, our loves, our fears, questions, and revulsions.

Our memories link us with the world of nature. They remind us how connected we are with the elements that form our planet—air, fire, earth, and water—especially water. We're rocked in fluid before birth, and water makes up 70 percent of our adult bodies. Water is a primary conductor of our body's intelligence, and of elemental, cosmic intelligence. No wonder so many women's memories of sex and spirit resonate with fluidity and flow. "Warm waves washing over me, like a gentle ocean washing over my soul," writes an ISIS woman describing her most luscious sexual experiences.

Since so much of our body is composed of water, I was particularly interested when a healer friend gave me *The Hidden Messages in Water,* by Japanese physician Masaru Emoto. This remarkable book of photographs shows how water responds to human messages. When water received messages of love and gratitude, the ice crystals it formed were intricate and beautiful. But when the messages were about control or hatred, the crystals were gray and distorted, or they failed to form at all. Rather like my early upbringing, I thought. And like the backgrounds of so many women who've experienced control or violence in the name of sex.

These images of water dramatically demonstrate the workings of the universal mind: Our beliefs and messages literally create form. Consider how this is true of our sexual forms—harmony and flow or discord, ugliness, and denial. It's not that we simply react to messages and beliefs about sex. We may quite literally embody those messages and beliefs. We may *become* them. Granted, there are sexual situations we can't change simply by changing our point of view. But there are situations that can—and will—change when we shift the way we think about them.

And this is the ultimate lesson of the mental path of the ISIS Wheel. Simply being on the path in a spirit of respect, confidentiality, safety, and open-minded wonder can determine the form our sexuality takes. How we (and our partners) think, how we imagine, how we dream, how we remember can construct erotic experience as a positive and powerful part of our lives.

CHAPTER EIGHT

DOORS TO THE UNIVERSE

Your Spiritual Journey

ISIS WOMEN SAY sexual experience can open up "doors to the universe," a universe that includes vibrant light and color, intense feeling, and revelation. These doors may open to transcendent encounters with God, Goddess, Spirit, Higher Power—or whatever name fits your belief system. Or you may find yourself plunging deep into the story of your own life to discover the profound truths of your own creativity and resilience. Either way you feel one with yourself, with your partner, with nature, with all that is. This is the spiritual path of the ISIS Wheel. On this path all's right with your world.

Our spiritual journeys wake us up. They delight us, they inspire us, they can transform our lives. Women speak of increased energy, power, and pleasure—more positive attitudes, more honest relationships, clearer purpose. A thirty-two-year-old ISIS woman from Alabama says connecting sex and spirit liberates her from the doubt that sometimes assails her sexual pleasure. "I feel myself climbing upward, and when I reach the peak I'm released of any bad feelings, any bad thoughts. It's as though I've done no wrong, and I can start over again." A twenty-nine-year-old Nebraska woman writes of the strength and direction she receives from connecting sex and spirit.

I have experienced sex as a gateway to the soul—my soul, the soul I am making love to and God and all that is—including spiritual guides. By experiencing sex as a spiritual tool, I have grown strong in intuitive and telepathic abilities, and grow closer and closer to God. More one-ness with All and more power to open doors to create what I choose.

The word "spiritual" comes from the Latin *spirare,* which means "to breathe"—a process that's central to our bodies, our vitality, and our life force. We can't live without breathing. The spiritual ISIS journey doesn't mean turning away from your body, away from your senses. To the contrary. It means tilling your garden of earthly delights as thoroughly as you can. This is a paradox of course, and ISIS women often speak in paradoxical terms. They speak of the "divinity" of down-to-earth activities—a familiar smell, a whispered name, an intimate touch that inspires and moves them beyond the physical. They speak of heart-thumping excitement, and at the same time a peace that passes understanding. A fifty-year-old woman from New Jersey writes that connecting sex and spirit is "powerful enough to manifest joy through me and bring me to my knees at the same time."

In short, your spiritual journey is not an out-of-body experience. It's connected with physical sex, too—even hot, sweaty humping, as long as it's meaningful to you. Your spiritual journey is connected with all your ISIS paths. Think about your own most meaningful sexual experiences. Perhaps you've felt transported to divine realms—ISIS women speak of meeting God, Goddess, and countless nature spirits. You've probably also experienced emotional cloudbursts like falling in love. And some meaningful physical moments, like masturbating for the first time, or your first orgasm. And some of your most meaningful sexual experiences may be rooted in the slow details of intimacy.

How did you learn about connecting sex and spirit? Looking back, I can see that this connection was always there for me. It was at the center of my most generative choices, certainly for sexual partnership, and motherhood, even my choice of career as a therapist and researcher. But for most of my life there wasn't any language to affirm these experiences. I was a grandmother before I fully understood how intricately woven my physical desires were with what I felt was most precious and holy. I'm totally impressed by young women who already understand this and can articulate when and how they learned this truth.

Most ISIS women say they connect sex and spirit through relationship with their partners. Some say they've been aware of the connection from earliest memory ("I learned from the good, respectful, and sexy marriage of my parents." "I grew up on a farm and connected sex with birth, death, and so on."). Some became aware late in life (a fifty-five-year-old writes, "I discovered the connection when I was forty-eight"), and some as recently as "last week." Others say they're acutely aware of the connection even though they've never felt its full power. Others say they learned directly from their bodies. I love what a California massage therapist writes about her capacities for accessing what she calls life-force energy—and her wish for equal partnership:

> My explorations and experiences as an energy worker have brought me into contact with others who are as sensitive as I am. However, I have yet to experience a LOVER with my abilities. When I do have the pleasure of sharing on this level with my partner . . . well, Planet Earth will get the ride of her life.

SPIRITUALITY AND RELIGION
What's the Difference and What Do They Mean for Our Sexuality?

It's easy to confuse the terms "spirituality" and "religion." They're both about beliefs and values. They both suggest there's something out there that's more than physical, more ultimately satisfying than performance. There are major differences, though. Spirituality is about your personal beliefs and values. It concerns your relationships with human beings, nature, and divine presence as *you* experience them. Religion is an established system of beliefs and values about the divine; it involves cultural traditions and rituals, some of them literally carved in stone centuries ago. Your spiritual beliefs may shift over time. Religious doctrine is forever.

ISIS travelers are likely to meet both religion and spirituality on their journey toward the center, for rich connections weave through sex, spirit, and religion. These stem from pre-Christian religions, which worshipped the human body along with sun, moon, wind, rain, and other sacred mysteries of nature. Especially, they worshipped women's bodies and their magical cycles of blood and pregnancy and birth. To celebrate all this natural fecundity, sexual union was built in to early worship—sometimes to wild excess, as in Bacchanalian orgies and Celtic Beltane ceremonies with May Day bonfires and gluttonous mating. Lustiness was next to godliness—along with feasting, drinking, and dancing. Pleasure, orgasm, and ecstasy weren't sins. They were routes to the deity.

Some religions are still based on the idea that sex can be a path to spirit: Tantric Buddhism, Chinese Taoism, Wicca, and various indigenous practices. But even some of our major religions carry vestiges of the early sexual rituals. Candles and incense, wine, flowers, music, anointing with oil, laying on of hands—all these come from those pagan rites. We've adapted them into the Catholic Mass and Protestant Eucharist without ever acknowledging their pagan sexual roots. And here's the most interesting part—we've also adapted them into our customs of courtship and mating without ever acknowledging their spiritual connections. Many ISIS women do acknowledge the associations, though, and use them to bring spirituality into their sexual relationships.

I used to think we had no language to express the connections between sexuality and spirituality. Then I began to understand that ISIS women often use religious terms to express their sexual feelings. The flush of sexual ecstasy is "holy," "sacred," "a revelation," "a sacrament." They cry out "Oh, God!" in both churches and bedrooms the world over. The truth is, the scientific and locker-room language we have for sexual experience describes only a fraction of the whole picture—the performance part. The picture changes when women's voices are factored in, especially the voices of ISIS women.

How ISIS women see religion affecting their sexuality is also complex. The response can be negative: "I was afraid to be a sexual person because of all the rules laid down by the Baptist church." But it can be positive, too: "My deep religious faith has led me to know that sexual love is also sacred love." "My spiritual practice gives me the courage to work through the intensity of my relationships." "It's in orgasm that I've seen the face of God." A forty-two-year-old teacher from North Carolina was one of the very first women to respond to the ISIS survey. She braids all of these elements together in a small miracle of a poem about sexual-spiritual-religious communion. Notice that she begins with the word "breath"—the spirit of it all.

MIDNIGHT MASS

the breath
of life
flows back and forth
between us
as we pray in
near darkness
the door
slightly ajar
lines of yellow light
streaming in on
the pious

we dance
on cotton cloth
hymns sung behind us
before the offerings
in praise
of body
and spirit

being in bed
with you
is
receiving communion.

sips of water, wine
cleanse us
as we atone for
half-truths and old scars

BARRIERS TO CONNECTING SEX AND SPIRIT AND HOW WE OVERCOME THEM

"Man, Catholicism sure does screw up one's 'pleasure thoughts,'" writes a thirty-three-year-old Nevada woman who says she hasn't engaged in any kind of sex at all since she was twenty-two, when she kicked her drug and alcohol habit. "I do not even masturbate the way I've heard other women have because I feel so guilty and ashamed if I bring myself pleasure." My heart goes out to her. This is a kind of sexual paralysis I witness in countless clients who have sought help with low sexual desire or no sexual desire at all.

Guilt, shame, and desire problems can be part of the fallout from repressive religious beliefs—and much is written on the subject by both sex therapists and clergy members. But it's not only the church. In my years as a therapist I've learned that our whole society can function as an effective training program for "screwy pleasure thoughts." There's our culture's separation of the mind and the body. There's also sexual abuse, sexism, racism, homophobia, poverty, politics—you can add to this list by reading your newspaper almost any day. Include all the personal roadblocks we bring with us—too much work, too little sleep, too much distraction, too little time, too much alcohol, too little trust, and on and on. Not to mention relationship troubles, problems finding a partner, or disabilities that affect sexual performance and may focus us on our pain instead of our pleasure. All these add up to the lack of sexual desire women are bringing into therapy offices all over the country. Some call it sexual dysfunction. I call it disconnection of sex and spirit.

The amazing thing is that women heal from these disconnections—and not always through therapy. Some women leave their religions—they either walk away altogether or else find ways to worship that are more sex- and woman-positive. Some change their sexual orientation—straight women fall in love with women, lesbians fall in love with men. Partnered women enter periods of celibacy and discover *themselves* for the first time— "Omigod, I've been waiting for you all my life!" Unpartnered women finally connect with a compatible partner—"a loving, *conscious* partner who cares about me." Some women pray, some meditate, some masturbate, and some enter therapy. Some connect sex and spirit by working through their addictions on their own or in self-help groups.

For still others, healing from the disconnections seems to be a spontaneous, even magical process—through dreams, sudden visions, or hearing lyrical music of the spheres—(this is not a total fantasy; seismic studies have revealed that the hum made by the movement of the planets creates an actual "space symphony"). Some women journey to awesome shamanistic realms to find helpful spirit guides. A dear friend I regularly meditate with had an extraordinary vision that included an explicit instruction: She was told to connect with the "highest vibration" of everyone she met—that is, she was to contact the best in them instead of getting sucked into their negativity. This is a daunting feat. Try it yourself—especially while you're standing in an endless line at the post office or negotiating with your ex over child support. You may not always be able to change the situation, but you'll be able to change yourself. To connect with *their* highest and best, you'll have to contact *your own* highest and best. To do this, you'll have to breathe fully instead of holding in—*spirare*, the ISIS route to connection and meaning. So even in nonsexual situations, using your breath to connect with your highest vibrations can put you in the ISIS mood.

For some ISIS women, connecting sex and spirit is part of the long, grinding process of coming to terms with physical or mental disability—and this can be a significant step in learning to love themselves for the first time. A twenty-seven-year-old New Jersey woman writes of her struggle with Crohn's disease—a chronic life-threatening inflammation of the bowel. She calls her condition "embarrassing and painful," which is a vast understatement, for she says she's already undergone forty hospitalizations and nine surgeries to repair her damaged intestines. Yet her message is about hope and healing, and opening up her belief system.

> Not only do I not get out much, but I've been working on overcoming pain, loving myself, and my quest into consciousness. After several years of completely ignoring sex and pleasure, I'm now realizing it has a definite place in my healing process. Before I find a partner, I feel I need to be comfortable with myself first and learn to masturbate. I read a little of [Margo Anand's] *The Art of Sexual Ecstasy* and it stunned me, grossed me out, and excited me. I'm really looking forward to integrating sex and spirit and experiencing an orgasm for the first time. Right now I'm starting over and I've taken baby steps. I have to first change my entire belief system. I'm starting over—wish me luck. . . .

Some ISIS women say they've actually been able to use their negative experiences as a path to sex and spirit. A fifty-one-year-old abuse survivor from New Jersey speaks of finding the connection through nature:

> As a child I used to escape from sexual abuse by "disappearing" into nature: trees, rocks, the earth, etc. This formed the basis for an abiding sense of oneness with all of the earth, so my spirituality was sort of "built in" as a result of sexual abuse. After years of therapy I was able to experience the presence and joy of this union in the union of marriage. It was wonderful to bring it all consciously together.

The bottom line is that when you connect the dots between sex and spirit, be prepared to expand your whole self. Your sense of love, creativity, altruism, and even religious experience can grow exponentially. I am not trying to suggest that this level of sexual connection is the only way to clear negative energy and recover your personal wholeness. But clearly for some women it can be transformative. So I do suggest that you be open to the possibility and believe it when it happens.

How You Can Be a More Spiritual Lover

Sometimes the sex-spirit connection just happens, like a puff of wind blown in by the Good Witch of the North. You can't always depend on the winds, but there are numerous ways you can open yourself to the spiritual path of the ISIS Wheel.

Your spiritual journey doesn't have to mean approaching your sex life like an episode from *Mission Impossible*. You don't have to be a mistress of esoteric techniques. Access to this path is like access to all the other ISIS paths—listening to your heart, acknowledging the intelligence of your body, caring for yourself, appreciating your partner, and opening your mind to adventures. You don't have to have it all figured out ahead of time. Many of us come upon our spiritual awakenings with the innocence of a child.

(When my three-year-old granddaughter asked "What's an adventure Grandma?" I answered "It's when you don't know exactly where you're going." And I hope she has many adventures in her life.) So when you enter the ISIS spiritual path, you have a brave new universe to explore. Be prepared to venture into some unknown terrain, and perhaps beyond your comfort zone.

But don't expect sex to transport you to bliss every time. It won't. And it doesn't need to, because connecting sex and spirit can nourish you so profoundly—way beyond a "Didja come?" model of physical satisfaction. When you're on the spiritual path, the standards for sexual fulfillment don't depend on how you perform.

Your journey will almost certainly vary as you grow older, or as you start a demanding job, or commit to a new partner, or become pregnant, or have a baby, and on and on. Shifts happen, as they say, and it's a good idea to keep this in mind so you can determine what's right for you *now*.

Here are some suggestions for your journey on the spiritual path. If you have a partner, by all means talk about these together. If you find it difficult to bring up the subject of sex and spirit, try highlighting suggestions you like and asking your partner to read them.

Practice safety as erotic foreplay

Safety is important on the spiritual path, and it's crucial if you have a history of hurt or abuse. Wounds of the body are also wounds of the spirit. All the internal armor you had to develop in order to survive the past may be preventing you from feeling a full range of pleasure now. And tight armor can definitely keep you from connecting sex with spirit.

Physical safety is clearly important to prevent sexually transmitted infections or unwanted pregnancy. Check out the resource section for how you can find information about condom use and other safer-sex practices. But most ISIS women need more than physical safety. So build in plenty of emotional and spiritual safety as part of your unique sexual style. You may need to hear soft words and feel soft hands—reassurance and tenderness, prayer and meditation. You may need locked doors (if you're so inclined, you can think up opportunities for kinky excitement here). You may need to exorcise the spirits of your abusers from the bedroom—poof! (For hot tips, see chapter 16, on creating sexual ceremony.) You may need to reconnect with rebellious parts of yourself—like the little kid who's kicking and screaming at the idea of any sex at all. Give her a fun job, like playing with the massage oil. She may make a mess, but she'll keep herself entertained so that the rest of you can focus deeply on connecting with yourself and your partner.

Above all, accept your own needs for safe passage on the ISIS Wheel. Safety isn't just an avoidance mechanism to put off engaging in intercourse, which many people regard as the only "real" sex. It's necessary to help you build energy, allow more desire and pleasure into your life, and connect with spirit.

Make time, set the stage, and follow your bliss

It takes time to set the stage for spirit—this is not a "quickie," at least at first. You can strew your space with flowers to bring in the nature spirits. You can light candles and incense to bring in the fires of mystery and passion. You can fix special food and drink to whet your sensual appetites. You can sing, dance, play music, whisper words of love and comfort. Certainly you can exchange touch. These may sound like cliché props for the "hot summer nights" issue of a glossy magazine. But they're much more. All of these practices are also time-honored parts of spiritual and religious ritual—as outlined earlier. Chapter 16 offers many more details on how you can set the stage for spirit.

Speak your heart

Almost all ISIS women agree that sharing deep feelings is essential on the spiritual path. You may need to laugh, cry, bare your soul. And by all means break with your good-girl training by speaking up for what you want. Let your partner (and yourself) know all about your ravenous desire for meaning and connection.

It's important to be clear about how you communicate, even when messages come directly from your soul. So follow these ground rules to make sure your deep sharing leads you where you want to go.

- Use "I" statements: "I feel." "I want." "I am . . . ."
- Keep it positive. Offer liberal amounts of appreciation and praise—to yourself, to your partner, to the cosmos.
- Accept all appreciation and praise that comes to you (this can be tough for women who've been taught to put themselves down routinely, but get used to it. It's time to learn to tough it out).
- Keep it simple. Too much talk gets in the way of feeling and being. Remember the ancient Chinese saying, "Talk does not boil rice."
- Listen to your partner. Erotic connection is always a two-way street.

Unleash your "wild woman"

There may be times you crave an element of risk, surprise, or outrageous fun, especially if sex has grooved into a rut. Two-thirds of the women who answered the ISIS survey say letting go of control is crucial to connecting sex and spirit. So let your wild woman out of her cage every once in a while—as long as you can do so in an atmosphere of mutual safety and pleasure. Have you ever wanted to kiss as if these were the last lips on the planet? Or dress like a cavewoman? One woman says she and her husband made love as if they were animals and chased each other growling and gnawing all over the house one Saturday morning. This primitive, elemental connection filled her with power she didn't know she possessed. In that sense it was a spiritual breakthrough for her. And it was transformational for her relationship. It pushed the boundaries to the outer limits, and she and her husband were able to travel much farther than they'd imagined.

Jungle activities may not be your cup of tea. But this story is a reminder that "spiritual" is not all about messages from angels. It can also mean tapping the murky depths of your most forbidden desires, whether or not you decide to act on them. For plenty of playful ideas, look in Annie Sprinkle's book *Spectacular Sex*. It's a trove of wild-woman treasures. Tonight can be the night! Engage all your senses. Divine!

Nurture each other, but don't forget yourself

Most ISIS women are awesome sexual caregivers. But all of us can probably benefit from focusing some of that earth-mother energy on ourselves. It seems that every other woman I see in therapy yearns for her partner to care more fully and deeply for *her*. But she worries that she doesn't deserve it, or won't get it. When all's said and done, most women fear that they'll somehow lose command of the situation. Endless giving may be a way to maintain some sense of control in your relationships. But at some point this strategy stops feeling good. It can be both exhausting and self-defeating. Spiritual sex isn't about one-way giving. It's a relationship dance of all the ISIS paths—a dance of all your senses and emotions. A dance of give-and-take.

A forty-one-year-old travel agent from Alaska describes just such a dance when she allowed her husband to reach through her caregiver defenses:

> We awoke in the middle of the night and made some tea. He sat behind me with his legs around me, my hands resting on his knees as he brushed my hair and I told him a story from my life. I remember feeling absolutely perfect, at peace, calm and serene as he tenderly ran the brush through my hair, stroking my neck and patting the hair back into place.

Letting your partner care for you is an affirmation of trust. It can be deeply spiritual and deeply erotic.

Open yourself to love

An abiding quality for ISIS women is a willingness to love and be loved. Remember your first moments of falling in love? If you're in a long-term partnership, you may find that what connects sex even more poignantly with spirit is commitment, intimacy, and sometimes day-to-day ordinariness. In other words, the whole multicolored fabric of the life you've created together.

My friend and valued colleague Maril Crabtree has a wise and wonderful story about the long-term benefits of loving. She recently attended a retreat where she was asked to answer three questions about what she'll want to say when she's eighty years old: "What was my life about? What did I care about? What do I want others to know that I did with my life?" (Before you read what she says, try answering these questions for yourself. It's an opportunity for you to write your personal manifesto.)

Here's what Maril says. She assures me that every statement is based on sexual relationship "in the broadest and most universal sense."

WHEN I'M AN OLD WOMAN I WANT TO LOOK BACK AND KNOW THAT I . . .

- Created joy and love for myself and others
- Lived truthfully, authentically, with passion and compassion
- Lived as a friend to all who sought friendship, and as a lover to all who wanted to be loved
- Walked lightly upon the earth, willing to share my resources with other species
- Gave willingly and generously of my time and skills to help others
- Carried love within me as a precious jewel, never forgetting its value and its presence

Open sharing of experiences like these breaks the conspiracy of silence about the fact that sex and spirit are connected and have meaning for our lives. And that this is true whether we recognize it or not, and whether we name it or not. May your spiritual journey bring you sharing, and magic of your own making.

And now we move to the very center of the ISIS Wheel, where body, mind, emotions, and spirit meet.

CHAPTER NINE

ECSTASY, MYSTERY, AND MAGIC

Your Journey to the Center

HOW VAST IS THE landscape of sexual pleasure? More vast than we know, for much of it remains unmapped. It lies in the realm of ecstasy, mystery, and magic, the realm where all paths flow into a unified whole. Here you are able to expand love, creativity, altruism, even religious experience. You open to energies beyond yourself—to nature and divine presence, to karmic lessons and prior lifetimes. Orgasm becomes a melting and merging into the cosmos—not a loss of your body and identity but an expansion of them.

ISIS women write about coming face-to-face with God, hearing celestial music, inhaling the breath of Shiva, conversing with the Great Goddess, cavorting with kundalini energy—a fundamental source of erotic power—and merging into an all-enveloping oneness that feels like making love with the universe. A forty-seven-year-old Idaho midwife writes of total identification with the universe, as if she is being *of* the universe, and actually *being* the universe itself:

I have, in the last two years, discovered sexuality to be a doorway to amazing cosmic experiences—experiences of oneness, not with my partner so much as with the universe—becoming light, a starry night, an ocean of love, pleasure itself. I feel altered—grounded, very peaceful and relaxed for days afterward.

Like so many ISIS women, she's describing an altered state of consciousness. I prefer the term "awakened state of consciousness," because this suggests an exquisite awareness rather than merely a quirky sidebar to the usual definition of "normal." Mystics and shamans call this "non-ordinary" reality. This is the ISIS connection—in the very center of the ISIS Wheel. It's where sexual experience enters the uncharted territory of ecstasy, vision, mystical revelation, and sometimes a grace beyond words or understanding.

THE ISIS CONNECTION

All the ISIS paths meet in the Center. Some women experience the magic of the Center as primarily spiritual and creative, some locate it primarily within their bodies, some in their minds or emotions. I've often heard women use the term "ecstasy" to describe the power of the Center. For some women, ecstasy means love and nurturing—a soulmate, an empathic partner, a sense of deep connection with themselves. Others say it's a delicious limbo outside of clock time. For still others ecstasy means creating new human life—conception, pregnancy, childbirth, breastfeeding—generative acts that literally embody the spirit of sexual union.

If ecstasy means entering fully into the center of the ISIS Wheel, sexual magic means stepping all the way through the Center and entering an entirely new dimension. Alice in Wonderland, Dorothy in Oz. This is a dimension that opens our minds and transforms our lives. It's where sexual experience becomes alchemy. Entrenched beliefs about the material world fade—including the desire-arousal-orgasm model of sexual function. The landscape grows ethereal or fantastical. Colors brighten. Time and space ebb and flow like ocean tides. Symbolic shapes and gestures hold potent meaning. What may seem "unbelievable" or "incredible" in ordinary reality is utterly authentic in the magical realms where your physical experience merges with mind, emotions, and spirit.

In the Center, even the concept of sexual partnership can shift and change. Human partners may morph into luminescent beings, sometimes from another time and place. ISIS women encounter energy bodies and spirit guides that are beyond direct physical, sensuous, rational experience. Some identify these as Christ, Shiva, God, the hand of God, the eye of God, and the voice of God. Others identify them as Goddess, Isis, Kali, angels, trees, sun, moon, star-born ancestors, animal allies, or beings they recognize from prior lifetimes.

Encounters like these can stretch the bounds of credibility, especially when they're in the context of sex. But such encounters aren't exclusive to ISIS women. They appear in the psychological literature—in Jung's exploration of archetypes and in the studies of peak experiences conducted by transpersonal psychologist Abraham Maslow in the 1960s. They're in medical accounts of miraculous recoveries and faith healing. They're in the Bible—in the *Song of Songs,* where sexual desire is inseparable from the holy bounties of nature: "Thy breasts shall be as clusters of the vine" (chapter 7, verse 8). They're in the diaries of the cloistered love-mystics such as Saint Teresa of Avila, whose *Vida* includes accounts of her orgasmic unions with Christ and his flame-bearing angels. They're in shamanic chronicles of sexual encounters with animal, angelic, and mythical beings from the Amazon rain forests to the Siberian steppes. And increasing numbers of theologians legitimize erotic energy as a form of prayer that communicates directly with God—Rita Brock (*Journeys by Heart*) and Carter Heyward (*Touching Our Strength*) are two of the most eloquent. Their wonderful books are listed in the suggested readings.

How women make the ISIS connection varies. Specific suggestions and exercises follow as the book progresses. The bottom line is that anyone can get there. You don't have to have an advanced degree or belong to a special club—though the resource section will guide you to how you can join an ISIS Connection group or start your own. But there's no highway that's guaranteed to speed you straight to the promised land. And you can't will yourself there any more than you can will yourself to be in love, or enjoy the taste of aged goat cheese—something I for one have never been able to achieve.

My wise friend and mentor Kaye Andres says making the ISIS connection begins with "set and setting." What she means by this is preparing yourself, and setting the scene. The "set" is about centering yourself in any way you know how. It may be through breathing or moving your body. It may be through immersing yourself in nature. ISIS women say they also prepare themselves through prayer, meditation, dance, chanting, and singing. A musician from Austin, Texas, points out, "Our sexual times were just extensions, expansions of our spiritual practice." One ISIS woman says she had her first orgasm as a teenager singing in the church choir, though she never recognized that was what it was until years later. Other women describe making the ISIS connection by more specialized means, such as shamanic drumming (described in chapter 19) or sounding the chakras (described in chapter 14).

If you're like most women who've talked with me, you don't need to develop a repertoire of erotic exotica (though don't let me stop you if that's your thing). ISIS women say that sexual magic can arise from the most "ordinary" or "routine" experiences, too.

LESSONS OF THE CENTER

Profound lessons may be embedded in your trip to the Center—a by-product of so many layers of connection. The lessons may be about expanding the spectrum of colors that our sexuality exudes, to borrow a phrase from my insightful colleague Patti Britton, author of *The Art of Sex Coaching*. Many of the lessons are about enjoyment and bliss—ISIS women speak of nirvana-like states composed of pure love. These are lessons you won't hear about in the physiological models of sex, where sexual experience is limited to predictable events you can count and measure.

The lessons of the Center can have their rocky patches, too. For one thing, there's the danger of becoming so attached to the kinds of feelings that arise there that you seem to need that degree of intimate connection all the time—and if you don't get it right away, you're gonna die! The psychological and pop-psych literature has words for this kind of chronic neediness, none of them pretty. These words include "hooked," "addicted," "dependent," "sexually compulsive," "nymphomaniac," "women who love sex too much." They all smack of pathology, and specialists have made a lot of money developing therapies and drugs to make them go away.

Mae West said, "Too much of a good thing can be wonderful." And I tend to agree with her—if you're able to drink in the feelings and savor them so that they enrich your life. In my sex therapy practice I've found that when people feel like bottomless pits of need, they may never have learned to contain their good feelings, so they require a degree of sexual affirmation that rules their lives—and their partners' lives, too. It may not be that they don't have enough sex, it's that they're not enjoying it enough. They're like leaky buckets. As soon as good feelings flow in, they flow right out again. Buddhist tradition sees this state as part of the human condition of suffering, or samsara, and points to the interesting image: the "hungry ghost"—someone who eats and eats and is never satisfied. Dante, in his *Divine Comedy*, places insatiable lovers in the second circle of hell, trapped in a violent storm, never to touch each other again.

If sexual neediness is part of your story, you don't have to stay stuck in samsara or hell. You can learn to fill yourself up. Many exercises in this book will guide you how to recognize good sexual feelings and breathe them fully into all parts of your body, mind, and emotions. This not only feels wonderful, it can also free you—and your partner—to enjoy sexual energy without having to act on every sexual feeling you have. Sometimes it's really that simple. I've found that the ability to acknowledge and contain pleasure in this way can help dissolve many a so-called "hyper" dysfunction or disorder.

But if a constant need for sex feels as if it's controlling your life and/or your partner's life, it may be time to seek professional help. Begin by talking with your partner, of course. Then consider some combination of spiritual guidance or sex therapy. Suggestions are listed in the resource section.

What the Center Is Like and What to Do Once You Get There

When ISIS women describe what the Center feels like, a kind of cosmic coherence shines through their stories. There are certain experiences that appear again and again. Three words stand out when women speak about the Center: *connection, meaning,* and *transformation.* These are not qualities you can count or measure—they belong to what Carl Jung calls the "irrational facts of experience."

You may not experience these all at once, but you may feel some of them, or some that are like them. Or you may have other experiences that are uniquely your own—you don't have to limit yourself to experiences on this ISIS list. The important thing to understand is that there really is such a thing as an ISIS connection—and that you can have it. Allow yourself to be fully present. Breathe. Believe it. Enjoy it. Remember it—that way, you bring the essence of ISIS home with you.

ONENESS AND CONNECTION

In the Center, you perceive everything as connected. You, your feelings, your life, your death, and your rebirth. You sense that you're aligned with the natural forces of the cosmos. I love what a fifty-six-year-old artist from Waialua, Hawaii, writes about this sense of merging with the universe— during sex with her husband, and later while masturbating. She describes "spontaneous experiences of transcendence" that intensified her awareness of herself and her relationship to the world. It was as if she had gone or been "elsewhere." Her husband called it "sexual fireworks," but her experience ventured well beyond an earthly blaze.

> Well, I *was* the fireworks. I felt as if I'd exploded into the Universe, and simultaneously "I" was also the Universe—exploding. I never thought of that again until a solo experience, which again blew me into a million fragments of light, then exploded me into some kind of divine, all-encompassing Light of Oneness and "I" was the All-and-the-Everything. With this remembered event, I just knew that "Something" exceptionally meaningful had happened again, and I didn't know what. But there indeed was "Something" here worth investigating and exploring deeply.

This sense of oneness is the blissful *unio mystica*, named by Western mystics—and it's attainable right in your own bedroom. *Hakuna Matata!* When you return to everyday life, I encourage you to bring this sense of harmony back with you. When you do, you may notice that the energy around you shifts. Women who've experienced this phenomenon say that people around them stop arguing and start smiling. Coworkers ask them if they've had a makeover. How good is that?

Direct experiences of God and the cosmos

Christian mystics speak of sacred light. Jewish mystics speak of Shekhinah. Shamans speak of spirit guides, guardian spirits, and power animals. ISIS women speak of intimate communication with divine beings. All signify that we are a part of cosmic oneness. A survivor of teen sexual abuse, now in her fifties, says she learned about the many faces of sex and spirit through the loving presence of an angel, who appeared for many weeks as a pillar of light. This being of "pure love" taught her that everything is related, including sex and spirit. "I was ready," she says, "having totally opened my heart to love. This experience is up there with giving birth to my babies and receiving true love from my parents."

You may not be able to see angels; you may not even want to see them. But her description lines up with many stories of abuse survivors who speak of spirit guides and angelic beings who come to help and teach them. The important thing is for you to recognize experiences you may have of God and the cosmos, in whatever form they take. The experience may be as simple as finding a feather in your path that delivers a message about lightening up your sexual interactions. Or seeing a rainbow that reminds you to look at the full spectrum of your experience.

Love and altruism toward the world

Experiencing the oneness of the Center is literally being in love. "Swimming in an ocean of love," one ISIS woman says. Another woman writes that she was transported to this state when she felt how deeply her partner looked into her eyes and told her how much he loved her: "That was enough to blow me into another dimension."

This is not the kind of love that means angst-ridden attachment—Is this "true" love? Should we marry? Divorce? Have a baby? Yadda, yadda. In place of all these head noises you feel a tenderness for all of humanity. You understand that the universe is ultimately benevolent. More than that. You understand that the universe is composed of love itself. You have a sense of being deeply satisfied, content, and renewed. Loved. In Love.

A forty-three-year-old graduate student describes the warm release she felt when she was finally able to let go of her belief that "sex was dirty and God wanted no part of it"—even within marriage. She says her many experiences of deep connection—both with herself and with her partners—revealed a loving, sex-positive universe. This consciousness permanently transformed her negative beliefs.

> The presence of all-encompassing love seems to flow through me, and if I am with someone, it seems to flow back and forth between us and this presence. Like a deeply spiritual experience, it takes me out of myself while at the same time making me intensely aware of the whole being that is me, and of a loving, embracing presence.

Heightened meaning

Reaching the Center is a peak experience and it's natural to attach a great deal of meaning to it. It may change the course of your life and open you to your fullest potential. It may strengthen your relationship. If your partner has a similar experience, this can be a great bond for you both. But attaching meaning can have a downside, too. Some women don't understand their journeys to the Center. They feel scared and overwhelmed. Their partners may not understand these journeys either. Sometimes it helps simply to know that experiencing the Center is extraordinary, and that you're not alone in your feelings.

Understanding and purpose

When you're in the Center, there can be a sense of omniscience, of knowing it all, of seeing it all unfold—and this sense can last well beyond the experience. This isn't some megalomaniacal mind trip, as if sex has handed you the revealed truth and everyone else should follow you mindlessly over the cliff. Instead, it's experiencing the ancient principle that thought creates form. You've met the infinite mind. You've cleared your anxiety and doubt, for an instant, anyway—which can be an eternity in the parallel universe of the Center. This knowledge helps you exude an inner knowing even if your workaday life may be in turmoil.

I'm impressed by the wisdom of an eighteen-year-old student from Johnson City, Tennessee. Her journey to the Center led her to understand the sacred and shapeshifting relationship between nature, spirits, and human beings—and led her to connect with the earth as a lover:

> I felt good and alive. I dreamed of beautiful natural scenes. In that dream I saw the earth as a woman. She was beautiful and radiant in a sense I would call divine. In my dream, we mutually caressed and aroused each other. When we both mutually reached orgasm I saw her face and the universe at the same time. I saw her as the beauty in every person, a very spiritual and sexual step for me.

Awe and wonder

Being in the Center fills many of us with amazement—and a longing to return to the sweetness after we come back to our everyday realities. The woman quoted above describes her response to the alchemical exchange she experienced with her partner:

> The barriers, the resistance, the pettiness are gone for that moment. There is a feeling that reminds me of what it must be like when two electrical charges unite to form an atom. I can always tell when I have had such an experience, because for some time afterward I seem to have

a heightened awareness of everything around me, including what I am feeling.

I've often worked with clients to help them incorporate this sense of awe and sweetness into their everyday lives. There's a simple breathing exercise you can try if you want to extend your own wonder-ful moments.

Breathe in, breathe out.
Breathe in awe, breathe out sweetness.
Breathe in sweetness, breathe out awe.

Let sweetness and awe spiral through you like strands of DNA. Notice how your body feels. Notice how you feel. Awesome.

Beauty

In the Center you are beautiful. Your movements flow. Your hair is glossy, your skin is smooth, and your voice pours forth like pure, sweet honey. When you return to everyday life, you get to bask in the afterglow of all this beauty. Everything looks vibrant. The trees shimmer. Your house shines. Everyone you meet radiates health and awareness. I'm reminded of the poignant Navaho prayer, "I Walk in Beauty":

> Beauty before me.
> Beauty behind me.
> Beauty above me.
> Beauty below me.
> Beauty all around me.

This prayer holds powerful medicine. Sometimes I chant these lines over and over to remind myself that I really do live in beauty even when the day's news makes me want to cry. The more you repeat this prayer, the more it is likely to open your heart and connect you with the center of your own experience. And the more filled with inner beauty you'll become.

Transformation

When you reach the Center, you may experience a kind of amazing grace that permanently changes how you perceive your life. You cannot explain this to yourself or anyone else through a process of logical thought. This kind of grace is one of Jung's "irrational facts." The effect is that your ordinary, everyday experience becomes different—larger, more meaningful, more mind-blowing. The idea of magical transformation through sexual interaction is not new. Psychologist Jenny Wade points out that it goes back to the oldest document we know of, *The Epic of Gilgamesh*, which graphically describes the taming of a dreaded monster through sacred sexual union with a woman.

ISIS women report that the transformative effects of sex can be dramatic. A twenty-five-year-old medical assistant from Trenton, New Jersey, writes of a supernatural experience while she was meditating with candles, incense, tribal music—"the works," as she puts it. Here she was visited by the "Higher Powers" in a way that recalls the sexual ecstasies of Saint Teresa.

> I began swaying to the beat, allowing the music to flow through me, and there was a cool breeze blowing almost from nowhere, and I could feel my body begin to tingle. I felt like I was flying and as if there was someone with me—touching me, caressing me, entering me. As the beat strengthened, so did these feelings of ecstasy, until the point of climax, when I began to exit meditation slowly, quietly, and peacefully. That was the point when, without a doubt, I felt the Higher Powers within me. And I have never been the same. I knew I had been changed spiritually and sexually forever! And that the two [sex and spirit] definitely walked hand in hand.

Letting go of control, letting go of ego

Letting go is part of the transformative lesson of the Center. This doesn't mean submission, knuckling under to a dominating force—most of us have already done that kind of knuckling, and don't want to go there again. In the Center, letting go means surrender, letting go of preconceived ideas, past negativity. It means flowing with what's happening rather than trying to resist it or push it one way or another. It implies trust that you're loved and cared for. In the Center, you don't have to be the stage manager or the placator. You don't have to provide the meals or clean up the mess. Some women find this hard to hear, but there's a potent payoff to letting go. "I learned I'm a human *being* rather than a human *doing,*" says one ISIS woman. You can do it too. I am woman: hear me surrender.

Surrender also means a degree of ego loss. This doesn't mean you lose your sense of self. Rather, it means you're able to move through the boundaries that keep you separate from the powerful energies of the universe. Letting go of your ego in this way can be both freeing and empowering— because you don't have to whip yourself into performance mode or be afraid of doing it wrong. You can be totally in the present. You can trust. You're *there.* And knowing there's a Center, you know there is a "there."

Suddenness and/or synchronicity

You may find yourself "there" before you know it, instantly transported from the world of physical pleasure to a place of magic and wonder. And on your return you may find some delightful synchronicities in your life. Uncanny things happen. People materialize as if you've summoned them simply by thinking about them. Opportunities magically open. A forty-one-year-old ISIS woman writes of the synchronicities she experienced with her first long-term partner, which, she says, went way beyond how other people talk about their relationships: "We would be able to 'find' each other at will in the town we lived in—without planning it. It was as if we were part of some larger energy or intelligence. There was a grace and beauty as well as calm and energy at the same time about it."

Luminescence

Hundreds of ISIS women have told me that their deepest and most meaningful sexual experiences are filled with light. The brilliant quality of this light is typical of spiritual revelation, and it's one of the signatures of the

Center. A thirty-one-year-old clerk from Ontario, Canada, describes the luminous space she once entered during lovemaking.

> It was as if I was bathed in warm, golden light—light so bright I could see it through my closed eyelids—and an intense sense of oneness with all of creation, a deep peacefulness and understanding in my soul—a tremendous sense of being centered—in myself, in my marriage, with the Goddess, and in the world and universe.

The transformational quality of this light may not always be peaceful. Sometimes it's explosive. It may suddenly break through during orgasm, or it might actually be the orgasm itself. (One woman speaks of "lightgasms.") Explosive light is also part of the paradoxical nature of the Center. The overall feeling is transcendent and holy, yet every cell in your physical body may be pulsing with sensation and panting for more stimulation. The overall feeling is unity and connectedness, yet you may feel blown into "a million fragments," like the artist from Hawaii. Perhaps the part that's blown is the rigid belief system about what sex should be, and that's what allows the ISIS transformation.

My colleague Maril Crabtree writes of bringing this transformational light back into everyday life and out into the open. She describes how she uses it in the ISIS Connection groups she conducts in Kansas City (see contact information for these groups in the resource section).

> We brought the light into our space through meditating. Then each of us bent down as if we were in a running stream and began to "wash" each other from head to toe with the gold energy-light. Over and over, we scooped up this magical energy and smoothed it onto each other's heads, shoulders, torsos, and feet. We laughed and smiled as if we were temple goddesses having a romp in a natural spring.

Timelessness

In the Center hours may go by. Or half a minute. Past and future may merge. Clock time becomes irrelevant. ISIS women describe this in a variety of ways. A fifty-eight-year-old speech pathologist from western Massachusetts writes, "Time stood still and our souls blended together into a perfect flow." "Completeness and floatiness," says a seventy-one-year-old designer from Santa Rosa, California.

My healer friend Reva Seybolt has a clock in her office that says, "Time Flies and So Can You." I like that sentiment a lot. To me it says you don't need to stay stuck in one reality. Once you let go of the concept of linear time, you can allow yourself to travel in two or maybe many realities at once. This kind of transformational "knowing" can expand your vision of sexual truth beyond what you may have learned from your doctor, clergy person, or even your partner, and locate it in your own ISIS experiences.

Movement—the sense of being on a journey

As you go into the Center or through the Center, your energy field changes, and you can feel as if you're being whirled in space. In a sense, you are. The energy in the Center is different from our ordinary street lives, and you can experience a sudden shift to feeling lighter, more mobile, more refined. Your mind opens up. Your heart expands. Your body's tissues pulsate with nutritive energy. Chinese medicine calls this energy *ch'i*. In India it's *prana*, in Hawaii it's *mana*. You may feel as if the earth moves. But it's actually you who are in motion.

Spontaneous healing

When the sexual frequency you enter is fine enough, you may enter a kind of antibiotic sphere where diseases cannot live, whether they're physical, emotional, spiritual, or mental. This is part of the transformative character of the Center. A striking example of spontaneous healing is described in chapter 5—a photographer's chronic heart condition disappears as if by magic once she reconnects with the warm sexual attentions of a childhood sweetheart.

Although spontaneous healing has its obvious benefits, it can create a special problem of its own: It can outrun your belief system. Exactly this occurred for the ISIS photographer. She says it made her feel "crazy," and she refused to tell her cardiologist that sex was part and parcel of her cure because she was afraid *he* would think she was crazy. In fact she continued feeling crazy until she heard similar stories from other women. The point here is that there's more to the healing power of sex than we can possibly know through so-called evidence-based medicine. So it's important to be open to the possibilities in your own life and to trust them. While a growing literature of mind-body healing affirms that satisfying sex can contribute to your overall health, reports about spontaneous sexual healing are rare. We need to legitimize it as part of sex "magic" and let each other know when it happens. As one ISIS woman puts it, "Maybe everyone is just polite—keeping quiet about this. When I first started experiencing it I thought, 'My God! Why didn't anyone tell me about this?!'"

Ability to perceive auras and other energy fields

Reaching the Center may reveal subtle abilities you weren't aware of. Or it may heighten abilities you're already using. You may suddenly see auras— the colored energy fields that surround our bodies. Chapter 14, on the chakra system, offers ways you can balance these energy fields to enhance your overall health and sexual health. ISIS women also report being able to hear music that's beyond their sensory hearing—some believe this is the hum made by the movement of the planets, some believe it's the sweet singing of angelic choirs. Women also report clairsentience—this is the ability to map other people's feelings in one's own body. New lovers do this automatically, as if they're tuned in to each other's channels. So do new mothers. They know instinctively—"in their guts"—what their babies' crying means. I believe many therapists do this automatically as well, and use it as an effective way to feel what their clients are feeling. It took me years to trust this ability in myself, though I always check my intuition with my clients' perceptions of what's happening for them.

The important thing to acknowledge is that reaching the Center can open your extrasensory perception in many ways. If you want to develop your intuitive abilities, you can search out workshops and trainings at the personal growth centers listed in the resource section.

Reexperiencing prior lifetimes

At the Center—where body, mind, heart, and soul meet—it is possible to feel transported to another time and place. You might see the embroidery on a toga or taste the musky juice of a pomegranate. You might meet your lover and soul mate—not in Jersey City or Minneola, where you live today, but in the agora in ancient Athens, or the temple of Karnak in ancient Egypt, or the grasslands of pre-Columbian North America.

Women who have had such experiences find they can give great meaning to their present relationships. It's possible to use them as a kind of Rosetta stone to help decipher present relational patterns, and to affirm the mystery and holiness of sex. A fifty-three-year-old minister from Newburgh, Indiana, describes her long-term relationship with "the man God had designed for me to live my life with." She writes that they'd felt drawn together by "destiny" after recurring memories of previous lifetimes they shared. On a lighter note, a forty-two-year-old interpreter from Santa Rosa, California, describes a sexual encounter that triggered a past-life memory in the gun-toting Wild West:

> I could hear the music playing from the saloon and the swinging doors flapping as I looked down the boardwalk, up the dirt street in the old Western town. I saw this handsome man [my partner in this lifetime] with black hat, black attire, and black horse coming into town. He pulled his horse to a stop [and] hitched the reins onto the post. He got off, and with all my glory I knew we were in love. He stepped onto the boardwalk and—*clink, clink*—I could hear them shiny silver spurs as he walked my way. We embraced. That was it.

What is striking about this experience is not only the wealth of detail—she also mentions a poke bonnet, French curls, and a twirling parasol—but that her boyfriend, as he later revealed, was simultaneously recalling the same events while they were making love:

> I really didn't recognize it until the next day. My boyfriend said, "Hey baby. Last night was really good. It was like back in the good ole West-

ern days." I was shocked. To this day I can still hear the *clink, clink* of those spurs.

Whatever your experiences of the Center may be, please don't regard them as goals or achievements for you to replicate or surpass, though it can be a temptation in this culture of the four-minute mile and seven-foot high jump. The important thing for you to understand is how they are useful to your life. What patterns do they reveal? How can you do more of what feels good and right? How can you change what doesn't work well for you? As this book progresses, you'll see how women integrate their ISIS experiences.

Litany of the Center: How Women Describe the Indescribable

It can be difficult to find just the right words to describe the experiences of the Center, the sense of wholeness, of oneness, the feelings of acceptance, of love. Yet many ISIS women do find words. I've gathered a small bouquet of their words and phrases here as an offering to the Center. What emerges is a kind of litany. In many spiritual traditions reciting a litany of names is a way of bestowing praise and proclaiming value, of declaring that one name is not enough. Consider that Isis herself is known as Goddess of a Thousand Names. Here is the naming of the ISIS Connection:

TO THE CENTER
Giver of Breath, Bringer of Peace, Breather of Wholeness, Embracer of Intimacy, Source of Serenity, Source of Joy, Source of Power, Being of Love, Face of Love, Lover of Lovers, Union of Everything, Creator of Inner Light, Giver of Vision, Fountain of Passion, Glimpse of Heaven, Enveloper of the Body, Gateway to Spirit, Planter of Spiritual Seeds, Respite from Chaos, All that Is, The Great All—Love.

CHAPTER TEN

IS IT DYSFUNCTION
OR IS IT COSMIC SEX?

Mapping Yourself from Performance to ISIS

"Am I normal?" This is a haunting refrain from women who come to see me for sex counseling and therapy. What most of them mean by this is "How does what I do and think and feel compare with everybody else's sexual experience?"

This is a sticky question even beyond the religious and moral definitions outlined in chapter 8. The truth is, there's no real way of gauging the sexual habits of everybody else, though some sex surveys claim they can. Take the notorious statistic that 43 percent of American women are sexually dysfunctional. As we've discussed earlier, this figure is based on survey questions that never ask what sexual satisfaction *is*—so how can we possibly know how many of us are satisfied or not, or whether or not satisfaction has anything to do with sexual function?

What are the standards, anyway? Does "normal" mean a lot of people do it or think it or feel it? Or does it mean something that's okay to do even if just a few people are doing, thinking, or feeling it? Or is "normal" a set of moral mandates—where any deviance is wrong, bad, evil? Maybe it boils down to a question of who claims the right to make those kinds of judgments—physicians, clergy, politicians, forensic experts, Judge Judy.

At the beginning of the twenty-first century sexual normality is still largely measured against the old Masters-and-Johnson performance model—physical arousal, intercourse, and orgasm. If this isn't what "does it" for you, you're left pretty much having to guess at what normal is. And if you're like most of us, you worry about it. Only the bravest of us are willing to admit we might be out of step. There can be nasty consequences for any deviation from the perceived sexual norm. God forbid you should talk about integrating sexuality and spirituality. Even some angels may fear to say they go there.

How do you find out what's normal sexual experience for your own life? I've found it can be extremely helpful to explore the differences between the performance model of sex and the ISIS model as a step toward making your own assessments about what's true for you. This chapter outlines three ways you can begin.

UP FROM "DOWN THERE"
From Performance to ISIS

The performance model is based on intercourse and physical orgasm. Intercourse is a natural act, as they say. You may be one of the many women who love it—the closeness, the sensations of enveloping your lover, the idea that you can co-create new life. If this is your story, you also have the satisfaction of knowing you're in the sexual mainstream. The problem comes when your partner's not a man or if intercourse isn't your thing. Or when a goal of orgasm becomes an on-demand performance that inhibits other kinds of sexual expression. Then sex becomes institutionalized into what I call the cultural missionary position, male standards on top—a big problem for many women.

My ISIS research shows that if you're in a strictly performance-based relationship, you're likely to experience a high degree of sexual constraint, fragmentation, and numbness. For instance, of the ISIS survey respondents who said spirituality is *not* necessary for sexual satisfaction, more than half reported having these emotional blocks.

In a performance relationship you're also likely to take some pleasure in controlling your partner—perhaps to compensate for feeling controlled yourself. Even so, strictly performance-model sex may work for you if you happen to be Jenny One-Note. But some ISIS women say they're frankly bored by intercourse—either because they don't feel very much on vaginal stimulation or because they find their partners to be emotionally closed, relationally clueless, or so locked into repetition that meaningful contact is out of the question. A thirty-four-year-old paramedic from Independence, Kansas (I'm not making this up), writes of breaking away from ten years in a performance marriage: "I am finally free . . . to discover who I am and what I believe and what gives me pleasure."

The ISIS connection is much more complex. As you've seen in earlier chapters, it opens us to a multidimensional world of body, mind, heart, and spirit. This ISIS world corresponds with the latest brain research, which shows that we're hardwired for such sexual complexity (I'll say much more about this in chapter 11). It also corresponds with the chakra energies and with time-honored Eastern spiritual traditions including Tantra, where sex and spirit are not separated from each other (more on these in chapters 12 and 13).

My research shows that if you're in an ISIS relationship, chances are you have a high degree of honesty and caring (true for some 80 percent of the women who answered the survey). Also a high degree of connection with yourself, your partners, and the divine (true for almost 70 percent of the ISIS women). If you have a history of sexual disappointment or abuse, your ISIS journey may help you restore your sense of self and pleasure—there are no numbers available on this, but scores of ISIS letters document this idea.

Clearly, performance and ISIS are two very different ways of looking at sexual experience. Does either of them feel like you? Perhaps you possess some characteristics of both. Below is an assessment chart to help you clarify where you are on your sexual path, and where you want to go. Other methods of assessment will follow. This one is especially for people who like to see their options lined up in rows.

It's important to understand that these columns represent the ends of a vast continuum. Most of us fall somewhere in the middle. And everyone's experiences are unique, so some of us fall off the edges of both columns. Still, it's interesting to see how the same experience can have different interpretations depending on which column you use to judge it.

PERFORMANCE AND ISIS
TWO MODELS FOR ASSESSING "NORMAL"

	THE PERFORMANCE MODEL OF SEX	THE ISIS MODEL OF SEX
Scope	One-dimensional—physical response	Multidimensional—body, mind, heart, and soul
Goal	Physical orgasm is the goal	Feelings and meanings are most nourishing and satisfying, especially over the long term
"Normal"	Based on the ability to achieve intercourse and/or orgasm	Based on safety, self-esteem, nurturing, pleasure, empowerment
Dysfunction	Inability to achieve intercourse and/or orgasm	Inability to connect with yourself, your partner, or the divine
Treatment	Behavior therapy, performance-enhancing drugs	Integrating your sexual responses, body, mind, heart, and spirit
Relationships and Gender Roles	Strict standards for sexual roles—usually based on power, double-standard Mars-Venus attitudes	Complex standards of sexual roles—usually based on feelings and meanings, equal power balances between men and women
Power	Men are more likely to initiate Performance	Women are more likely to initiate ISIS
Age	Sexual success and desire for intercourse decline with age	No "magic marker" at which sex is supposed to decline—ISIS sex may improve with age
Religion and Culture	Sexual rules and standards are often prescribed by religious and cultural traditions	Sexual rules and standards can be self-determined and negotiated between partners

For instance, using these two models, how would you assess the West Coast psychologist quoted below. Her story raises such interesting questions that I've sometimes brought it to my classes and asked students to argue both sides as an exercise in either-or judgment making. Is this woman describing sexual health or pathology? Is her experience sacred or blasphemous? You be the judge.

I have had sexual experiences in which I left my body, left the earth, was jettisoned out into space above the earth and looked back down upon it. During this experience I felt as if I touched the face of God and was one with God and all of nature. The feeling was one of ecstasy and exhilaration and a sense of otherworldliness. I believe the aspect of deep, committed, intensely devoted love and complete trust [in my partner] was what enabled me to completely let go and lose myself in the experience. Loving so completely somehow created an environment in which I transcended the physical and went beyond the bonds of being a mere mortal.

Begin by reading this passage out loud—and notice what you feel as you read it.

Next, apply the performance and ISIS models of sexual normality to the situation she describes.

Here's what my students found. Based on a performance model of sex, this woman is well off any of the physical orgasm charts. So is she "functional" or "dysfunctional?" A tough call, since she's patently enjoying herself and presents with no problem. But it's an easier call if you judge her strictly by the *DSM-IV* (the diagnostic reference manual used by mental health professionals). Her out-of-body experience with God could suggest that she suffers from dissociative disorder and/or delusional ideation. Verdict: She needs professional help.

What about assessing her by religious and cultural standards? In many conservative communities, it's not okay for God to appear as an object of sexual pleasure. Her quite biblical touching of "the face of God" could be labeled blasphemy because it's inspired by sexual stimulation rather than by religious devotion. Her God connection might be permitted if it were directed toward the sacrament of matrimony or the act of procreation. By mainstream standards this woman needs moral reeducation and perhaps intensive counseling.

If you base your judgments on an ISIS model of sexual experience, you get a different story. This woman's ability to move between the worlds is to be admired as multidimensional fluidity—the ability to travel all paths of the ISIS Wheel. Her direct communication with God is sacred, a manifestation of cosmic grace. Not only that, her experiences of God and sex are grounded in the contexts of "devoted love" and "complete trust" with her partner. These are highly valued by society at large, as well as by ISIS fans. Her ability to let go of control is something many women strive for—in fact it's a stated goal of many of my sex therapy clients. Her ISIS assessment: Wonderful! Will she appear on the morning news as a twenty-first-century role model? Probably not. So far, ISIS is an extracultural phenomenon.

This exercise only scratches the surface, but it helps us to appreciate the power of the models and standards we measure ourselves against—and to understand how subjective our conclusions really are. Once you set about judging how one person's sexual experience compares with anyone else's, you realize—news flash—*there are no objective criteria.* "Normal" is not an absolute. It depends on the sexual standards you choose as a basis for your judgments.

ASSESSING YOUR SEXUALITY
ON A CONTINUUM

Now let's see what happens to your sexual norms if you approach them as part of a continuum. The notion of conceptualizing sexual experience this way has a time-honored history in sexual science, by the way. Alfred Kinsey, the grand master of quantitative sex surveys, saw much of sexual behavior as well beyond either-or judgments. In his 1948 *Kinsey Report,* he famously created a zero-to-six scale to assess degrees of heterosexual and homosexual expression. For instance, if you identify as a "Kinsey-3," that means your sexual attitudes and behaviors are equally expressed with men and women.

An ISIS continuum of attitudes and behaviors ranges from purely physical sensation to spiritual enlightenment. On one end of the continuum are genital stimulation, intercourse, and physical orgasm. On the other end are transcendence and transformation. Most of our experiences fall closer to the middle than they do to either extreme. An exact balance between physical and spiritual would be an "ISIS-3."

I'm not suggesting that the ISIS scale is the ultimate in self-assessment. But it does require that you approach your sexual judgments with an open mind. It also allows a wide spectrum of self-reference. Here you get to think about your own experiences and place yourself on the scale rather than being placed there by an outside authority. In addition, it provides a way for you to include your spiritual and emotional responses, such as love, caring, and safety, as well as your physical responses.

The ISIS scale is open-ended. It allows you to acknowledge how your sexual experience may shift and change from one age frame to another, or from one partner to another. For instance, do you remember feeling unusually randy—or holy—when you fell in love? Or during your menstrual periods? Or during pregnancy? Or when you were nursing a baby? Or when you reached menopause? What happened to your sexual desire and expression when you experienced illness, affairs, abuse, or violence?

You can use this scale to chart all the interesting periods in your life—some people use it to take a full sex history of themselves. Note what you learn. Think of it as a linear way of walking the ISIS Wheel through your own sex history.

THE ISIS SCALE OF SEXUAL EXPERIENCE

0 —— 1 —— 2 —— 3 —— 4 —— 5 —— 6

Key

0 Physical, goal-oriented involvement only, with your self or with a partner. No perceived spiritual, emotional, or mental component. Satisfaction is expressed as physical, orgasmic release.

1 Intense physical response, with some emotional, mental, and spiritual aspects. Satisfaction is much more attached to physical orgasmic release than to emotional or spiritual meanings.

2 Physical aspects outweigh spiritual aspects, but with solid recognition of emotional, mental, and spiritual aspects. Satisfaction is somewhat more attached to physical orgasm than to emotional, mental, or spiritual meanings.

3 The ISIS fulcrum: an equal balance of physical and spiritual relationship. Physical sex is perceived as a path to the soul, to deeper relationship with self, partner, and the divine. Satisfaction is integrated among physical and emotional, mental and spiritual aspects.

4 Spiritual, mental, and emotional aspects outweigh physical aspects of sexual relationship, but with solid recognition of physical aspects. Satisfaction is somewhat more attached to emotional, mental, and spiritual meanings than to physical orgasm.

5 Intense spiritual connection, with some physical aspects. Satisfaction is much more attached to emotional, mental, and spiritual meaning than to physical orgasmic release.

6 Spiritual, mental, emotional connection only, with yourself, with a partner, nature, or the divine. No perceived physical component. Satisfaction is totally connected with transformational meanings, not body sensations.

Somewhere along the line it occurred to me that generalizing certain kinds of experience on a spectrum from the physical to the spiritual might help lift the stigma from our most culturally loaded terms and practices. Masturbation is a case in point. This is a term with such a toxic history that it's almost impossible to discuss it until you get past the moral outrage and bad jokes it engenders. Over the centuries, it's been associated with sin, sickness, insanity, and even the resignation of a United States Surgeon General, Joycelyn Elders. She was forced out in 1994, for recommending that sex education courses ought to inform young people that masturbation is a safe alternative to intercourse.

What happens if we assess our patterns of masturbating by using the ISIS scale rather than our deeply held prejudices? An "ISIS-3" might mean

"What's the big deal about touching your genitals for pleasure if you're also keeping yourself safe—plus touching your mind and emotions and deepening your relationship with yourself?" Thinking about our sexuality on this kind of multidimensional ISIS continuum can help us remove the stigma of the scary word and see our sexual practices in a new light.

WHAT THE MIRROR TELLS

Here's yet another way you can discover what "normal" is for yourself. It's a visualization exercise that can help you see your own authentic sexual response, which may or may not match the standards set by the culture.

One of the benefits of visualization is that it can lead directly into feelings and meanings. That is, it can fly beneath your left-brain radar that tells you "what you *think* you ought to be feeling," as one client puts it. So spend some time setting up this visualization. Before you begin breathe deeply, move your body, and let go of the tensions of the day.

If you want to receive all the benefits of this visualization, ask someone to read it to you—or record it in your own voice and listen to it. Then put on your favorite space music, lie back, and see what the mirror has to tell you.

Some women find it extremely helpful to keep a journal beside them to write down their observations as they occur. Post-Its also work well, and you can stick them right in the book and write the date on them for future reference.

I've also used this visualization in a group, where there's the added benefit of feedback from everybody else, which always enriches the stew.

Performance and ISIS: a visualization

Close your eyes and imagine that you're standing before two full-length mirrors. One mirror is labeled "Performance Model of Sex." The other is labeled "ISIS Model of Sex."

Begin by looking in the "Performance" mirror. In this mirror is reflected a "Performance You"—with all the traditions surrounding that, such as intercourse with a male partner, even if this isn't your style—and even if you're a lesbian. Let yourself imagine experiencing intercourse. Who's your partner. Be aware of him. How is it to have his penis inside your vagina? Feel what it's like to achieve the goal of orgasm. (In this model, orgasm is almost always seen as an "achievement.")

Whatever your experience, see yourself clearly in this Performance mirror. Notice the expression on your face. What are you wearing? Or not wearing? How are you moving your body? Or not moving? What kinds of memories emerge for you? Do you notice any bright spots? Or dark spaces? How do you feel as you gaze at yourself in this mirror labeled "Performance Model of Sex"?

Take another deep breath in . . . and let it out all the way. Ask the You in the Performance mirror to speak a word or phrase about what it's like to be in that place and hold those feelings. Speak this word or phrase out loud. If you like, open your eyes and jot it down in your journal.

Now close your eyes again and look into the other mirror. It is labeled "ISIS Model of Sex." In this mirror is reflected an ISIS You. See this now, even though ISIS may not be your sexual style. See yourself flowing like water. Feel your heart open like a flower. Move with the energy that surges through every bit of you. If you're with a partner, notice who it is.

Whatever your experience, see yourself clearly in this ISIS mirror. Your expression. Your clothing (or nakedness). Your movements (or stillness). Your memories. Any bright and dark places that appear in the mirror. How do you feel as you gaze at yourself in this mirror labeled "ISIS Model of Sex"?

Take another deep breath in . . . and let it all the way out. Ask the ISIS You to speak a word or phrase about what it's like to be in that place and hold those feelings. Speak this word or phrase out loud. If you like, open your eyes and jot it down in your journal.

Now ask the ISIS You and the Performance You to communicate with each other. What do they say? What do they do? Are they agreeing or arguing? Is there a place in the middle that they want to meet? Does their style of communication remind you of anything in your life? Speak your observations out loud and then write them in your journal if that feels right to you.

Were you able to see yourself clearly in each mirror? Are there any differences in how you experienced yourself in these two mirrors? What kind of feelings came up? Any surprises in what you experienced? Speak your observations out loud and write them down if you like.

Thank both these mirror images of yourself for appearing to you. And know that there's probably much more that each can tell you. You may find a whole story emerging as you begin to broaden your definitions of sexual experience and what it means in your life.

CHAPTER ELEVEN

HARDWIRED FOR ISIS

The Multidimensional Brain

YOU'VE HEARD WHAT women say about sex being more than a physical experience—about how it touches body, mind, heart, and soul. But where's the proof? What about some tangible evidence to show that the ISIS connection is real—that it's possible for any and all of us to integrate physical sex with how we think and feel and with what the whole experience means to us?

Our relationship with third millennial technology can address these questions—and more. Laboratory science is beginning to show that the routes to ecstasy, mystery, and magic run through the intricate miles of circuitry that transverse our brains. Whether or not we're consciously aware of our non-ordinary sexual responses, the potential for them is ever present. The advances in brain research can help you understand your journey on the ISIS Wheel from a scientific point of view.

Brain researchers and sexologists now have access to imaging devices that can give us new information about the workings of our brains and broaden our notions of sexual response. These include PET (Positron Emission Tomography) and fMRI (Functional Magnetic Resonance Imaging) scanners. Through these windows on the brain, researchers are discovering what most women (and yes, some men) have known from time immemorial: Sexual response is more than physical. It is a rich and complex experience that involves our whole beings. We are actually hard-wired to experience sex multidimensionally.

Since the late 1990s various imaging studies have demonstrated how our brains react to different kinds of sexual stimulation. For instance, when we're stimulated physically (stroking, hugging, kissing, nuzzling, licking, and general fooling around), the hypothalamus becomes especially active. Researchers can see it light up on the computer screen, an indication of increased blood flow to that area of the brain. The hypothalamus is part of the physiologic system of the brain that controls physical gratification along with hunger and sleep.

When sexual stimulation is primarily romantic (admiration, sweet-talk, heart-to-heart communication), brain images have shown that the amygdala becomes especially active. This is part of the emotional system of the brain that controls joy and surprise along with other feeling responses such as fear, anger, and grief. (If you've seen the 2004 movie *What the Bleep Do We Know!?*, you may remember the cartoon images of the "molecules of emotion" that dance through a boy-meets-girl flirtation scene.)

But all of the early brain-imaging studies on sexual response were conducted on men. No great surprise. Men are the default, the normative subjects for science. Most research of any kind is first focused on men, whether it concerns heart disease or sexual function.

WHAT ABOUT WOMEN?

During 2000–2001, sexologists Beverly Whipple and Barry Komisaruk broke the gender barrier in brain research. They conducted landmark studies at Rutgers and Wake Forest universities, the first to measure brain activity in women during vaginal and cervical self-stimulation and orgasm.

Their studies not only tell us about women's sexual response, they also demonstrate how significantly laboratory sex research methods have changed in the last few years. In the early 1990s I worked with this same research team to study whether women were able to have orgasms by imagery alone—without any touch—by focusing on their memories or fantasies ("thinking off," as one woman called it—you met her in chapter 7 on the mental path of the ISIS Wheel). We invited ten talented women (one by one) into Whipple's Rutgers University physiology laboratory and measured the correlations between the orgasms these women were able to generate through masturbation and the orgasms they generated through imagery alone.

In those days, which was an ice age ago technologically speaking, we relied on what women told us was happening, and backed up their self-reports through hookups that measured their heart rates, blood pressure, and pain levels. We also measured their pupil diameters, which are an especially accurate indication of the extent of physical orgasm. For this we used a pupillometer, an ophthalmic device that proved to be diabolically awkward in this context. It required that a woman lurch bolt upright mid-orgasm and stay absolutely still for thirty seconds with her eyes locked open, staring at an X we had pasted on the wall. Yes, we found that women can "think off" to experience physical orgasms we could count and measure. Not only that, they could do it under these stressful and sometimes hilarious laboratory conditions. (The whole story of this adventure is detailed in *Women Who Love Sex*, and the scientific findings were published in *Archives of Sexual Behavior* in 1992).

Fast-forward ten years and picture Whipple and Komisaruk now equipped with state-of-the-art technology, searching for how the brain might reveal some untapped secrets of woman's sexual response. They used PET and fMRI scans to record brain activity in yet another ten women who were curious and courageous enough to further science by attempting to bring themselves to orgasm in a laboratory setting.

Interestingly, Whipple and Komisaruk were not looking for sexual multidimensionality. They were actually looking to see if women's orgasmic responses to vaginal-cervical stimulation could bypass the central nervous system and travel through the vagus nerve—a separate nerve pathway that ranges throughout our bodies. Because they wanted to make a definitive statement about these sexual responses, they invited study participants whose vaginal-cervical sensory nerves could have no possible connection to the brain through the spinal cord. Five of the women in the study were therefore paraplegic, with transected spinal cords.

Whipple and Komisaruk's brain scans found that women's orgasmic response can indeed travel through the vagus nerve: the women with complete spinal cord injury had the same brain areas activated during orgasm

REGIONS OF THE BRAIN ACTIVATED DURING VAGINAL SELF-STIMULATION AND/OR ORGASM	
REGION OF THE BRAIN	WHAT THE REGION OF THE BRAIN INVOLVES
Hypothalamus	Hunger, sleep, physical gratification
Amygdala	Emotional response: fear, joy, anger, grief, surprise
Temporal Lobe	Religious ecstasy, spiritual experience, hearing
Midbrain reticular formation	Arousal, awareness
Midbrain central gray	Pain relief
Basal ganglia	Motor control
Cerebellum	Motor control
Hippocampus	Memory
Accumbens nucleus	Anticipation of reward and punishment
Anterior cingulate cortex	REM dreaming, primitive emotions, discernment
Insular cortex	Response to light touch
Paraventricular nucleus	Pair bonding

Adapted from a paper by Beverly Whipple, Ph.D., and Barry Komisaruk, Ph.D. Presented at the World Congress of Sexology, March, 2003, Cuba.

as the women without spinal cord injury. More importantly, to my way of thinking, their study also showed that *women's vaginal-cervical stimulation and orgasm activated multiple regions of the brain—and activated them simultaneously.*

These laboratory findings represent a major breakthrough in sex research. They provide the first truly objective data to support the idea that response to physical stimulation invokes much more than physical sensation—it may also invoke thoughts, fears, joy, surprise, memories, dreams, pain, pain relief, religious ecstasy, discernment, and anticipation of reward and punishment. Moreover, it shows that *all of these occur whether or not we're consciously aware that all of them are happening.*

These findings intimately parallel the responses to my ISIS survey, although ISIS women use decidedly nonscientific language to describe their multidimensional sexual experiences: "extraordinary," "luminescent," "mind-blowing," filled with "spontaneous healing" and direct access to "the core of universal love." The laboratory research affirms that sexual experience engages many of our brain's systems, and that these systems constantly communicate with one another to create a unified whole—physiological, cognitive, emotional, and spiritual.

In lay terms, brain science is telling us that sex is not the one-dimensional phenomenon so often indicated by other laboratory findings and by sex surveys. Sexual experience can also be unified, meaningful, and transformative—all the characteristics of the ISIS connection. An enormous complexity of events occurs that engages our bodies, minds, hearts, and spirits. Sometimes we notice them all, most of the time we don't. On this issue, sexual science and ISIS are finally walking hand in hand.

PART TWO

PATHS TO
THE HEART AND
SOUL OF SEX

CHAPTER TWELVE

WALKING THE
ISIS WHEEL

Making Your Way to More Meaningful Sex

You've read what science is saying about sexual response. You've read what many ISIS women say. But what about *you*? Perhaps you recognize your own experiences in these stories, or perhaps sexual multidimensionality is a new concept for you. Either way, this section provides further opportunities for learning what sexual experience might mean for your life. Below are suggestions for making the ISIS Wheel your personal map to more meaningful and satisfying sex—through exploring the pathways of your body, mind, heart, and soul. Feel free to adapt any of these suggestions to fit your situation. There's no one right way to walk the ISIS Wheel. Only you can determine which method works for you and which path to enter first. Here are some preliminary suggestions for how you might approach your journey:

• Trace the ISIS Wheel on page 33 with your finger or a pencil. You can write your perceptions as you move into and through each pathway, and even speak them out loud if this is your style. This method works well for *verbal* people, who find it useful to record information through taking notes and keeping journals.

- Find a space in your house where you can actually walk the ISIS Wheel. You can draw the ISIS Wheel in chalk or lay it out in string on your carpet. One woman traced it out in raisins on her big front porch. Move around in each pathway and let yourself experience what your body feels like as you move through each path. This method works well for *kinesthetic* people, who learn most easily through hands-on doing and through moving their bodies.
- Create the ISIS Wheel outdoors in nature so that you can connect with the elements—air, fire, earth, and water—along with all the helpful nature spirits who keep the natural world vibrant and colorful. Many ISIS women associate their most memorable sexual experiences with nature. Whenever space allows in my workshops, I bring women to a field or into the woods, or to a labyrinth where they can create their own ISIS paths, allowing their feelings to shift and change as they follow them into the center and back out again. (I've had my most profound personal ISIS Wheel experiences on beaches, where I can send feelings out into the ocean and know that the next tide will restore the sands.)

However you choose to walk the ISIS Wheel, notice your body—are you lyrical and flowing or tight and protective? Notice your breathing—is it full and energizing or shallow and constricting? Notice your voice—do you feel like singing or screaming, or perhaps whispering? What feelings or memories come to you? Call out names of any people from your past or present who come up for you as you walk the wheel. Make this a uniquely personal journey. Ask for inspiration and help. Express gratitude for what you are shown.

Explore each path for as long as it feels right. Then notice how you move from one path to another. Do you progress through the center of the ISIS Wheel? Or do you jump from path to path—for example from body to mind, perhaps unconsciously separating them? Do you find yourself wanting to stay forever in any of the paths? Or avoiding any of them? Or feeling stuck or uncomfortable in any of them? Notice how any of the experiences you have while walking your ISIS Wheel may be true in your life.

WALKING THE PHYSICAL PATH OF THE ISIS WHEEL

Below are some of the dimensions that ISIS women say describe their physical journeys on the ISIS Wheel. Which ones apply to you? What would you add to this list—or subtract from it?

- Skin hunger: The urgent lust for physical sensation.
- Genital stimulation and intercourse: Many women crave clitoral stimulation, some crave G-spot stimulation deep in the vagina, and some women feel complete and "filled" only with penis-vagina intercourse.
- "Outercourse" and extragenital stimulation: Many women are extremely aroused and even orgasmic on extragenital stimulation—touching all over their bodies; kissing, stroking, licking, blowing, nibbling, in any combinations. (A colleague once confided, "I don't know where on my body I'm not orgasmic; I need to be mapped.") See the Extragenital Matrix on pages 196–197.
- Responses to all the senses: Touch, taste, smell, sight, and hearing.
- Comfort, beauty, safety: Setting the physical scene for ideal lovemaking.

WALKING THE EMOTIONAL PATH OF THE ISIS WHEEL

Below are some of the emotional dimensions ISIS women say describe their sexual passion and heart-centered experiences. Which ones apply to your journey on the ISIS Wheel? What feelings would you add or subtract?

- Excitement: Anticipation, longing, joy, surprise.
- Self-esteem: The sense of being in right relationship with yourself, your partner, and the universe.
- Love: Tenderness, closeness, intimacy, yearning, delight in your beloved.
- Empathy: Appreciating your partner's feelings, wants, and needs as well as your own.

- Negative or scary feelings: Guilt, fear, hurt, rage, disgust, blame, and self-blame—these often coexist with joyful emotions and may need to be expressed in order to release the joy. Remember the ISIS woman from Florida who writes, "I wept, raged, laughed, prayed. It was one of the most healing moments of my life."
- Numbing and dissociation: Finding ways to turn off feelings when they become overwhelming.

WALKING THE MENTAL PATH OF THE ISIS WHEEL

Below are some of the mental dimensions ISIS women say describe their beliefs and messages, imagination, memories, and dreams. Which ones apply to your journey on the ISIS Wheel? Are there others you'd add or any you'd subtract?

- Positive messages: "I believe in myself." "Sex can be profoundly healing." "I can take charge of my own pleasure."
- Negative messages: "Good girls don't; they don't deserve sexual pleasure and aren't supposed to enjoy it." "I'm too fat, thin, hairy, ugly, loud. . . ." "I need a man to make me whole." "Sex and spirit are separate."
- Positive flashbacks: Memories and dreams of pleasure, beauty, comfort, longing, power; images, stories, and feelings that connect sex and spirit.
- Negative flashbacks: Memories and dreams of pain, control, abuse.
- Mystical metaphors: The understanding that sexual energy can connect us with nature and divinity.

WALKING THE SPIRITUAL PATH OF THE ISIS WHEEL

Below are some of the dimensions ISIS women say describe the "divinity" of down-to-earth activities on the spiritual path. Which ones apply to your journey on the ISIS Wheel? Are there others you'd add or any you'd subtract?

- Transcendence: Waking up to dimensions beyond those you can perceive with your five senses.
- Profound truth: Tapping into your own creativity and resilience.
- Visions: Extraordinarily vibrant light and color along with revelation of "unseen" dimensions, such as the structure of the universe or the face of God.
- Peace that "passes understanding": Willing surrender to a benevolent, life-affirming higher power.
- Ritual and ceremony: Appreciating the holiness of pleasure.

Walking to the Center of the ISIS Wheel

Below are some of the dimensions ISIS women say they experience in the Center—the sense that sexual energy is powerful enough to change their minds and hearts, and sometimes even the way their bodies function. Which ones apply to your journey to the Center? Are there others you would add or any you'd subtract?

- Unconditional love: Being fully in the energy of an all-encompassing loving, embracing presence that's beyond you and your partner.
- Meaning and understanding: Instantly knowing the purpose of life, and that you are part of a divine plan.
- Timelessness: Moving outside clock time; a sense that past, present, and future are all contained in the present moment—which can seem like forever.
- Boundarylessness: Moving effortlessly through physical, emotional, mental, and spiritual space; the ability to merge with (and even shape-shift into) trees, rocks, animals, nature spirits, heavenly deities, and other life-forms.
- Memories of prior lifetimes: A sense of being transported to another time and/or place.
- Transformation: Permanent change in how you perceive your sexual experience and your life.

CHAPTER THIRTEEN

WALKING THE ISIS WHEEL WITH YOUR PARTNER

Creating Paths to Intimacy

As ISIS STORIES SUGGEST, there are many ways to deepen the intimacy in your life, whether you've chosen to be in a conventional marriage or one of the many partnership variations available to us today. Below are suggestions for enriching your present sexual partnership—or the partnership you hope you have one day.

DISCOVER WHETHER YOUR RELATIONSHIP IS "PERFORMANCE" OR "ISIS"

The performance model of sexual relationship is characterized by one-dimensional physical response. The ISIS model is characterized by the feelings and meanings that nourish your whole being. These models are outlined in chapter 10—and they can serve as a springboard for discussing the values you and your partner live out in your own lives. One benefit of discussing your intimate relationship in terms of "performance" and "ISIS" is to keep you focused on the issues that concern you rather than diverting your conversation onto other highly charged topics, such as gender differences ("All men want is intercourse . . .") or appearance ("If you'd only lose a little weight . . .") Performance and ISIS differences aren't always drawn on gender lines. They can also surface when your sexual partner is a woman.

Which performance and ISIS aspects of sexual experience do each of you respond to? Are there aspects you feel are especially relevant to your own relationship? Do you both agree on all the aspects? Talking about these ideas and questioning each other about them can lead to a deeper understanding of both your partner and yourself.

Be sure you follow these basic guidelines for good communication:

- Turn off the TV and telephone, and find a time when you're not exhausted and can protect yourselves from interruption.
- Speak from your own feelings: "I feel . . . ," not "You make me feel," or "Everyone knows . . ."
- Allow each other equal time, make eye contact, and listen respectfully.
- Make a specific time to continue your discussion if you don't feel totally in agreement about how you approach sex.

To help you begin your discussion, here are some of the conditions that many ISIS women said helped them to have the most powerful and meaningful sexual experiences—which ones apply to your life?

- Being in love
- Sharing deep feelings
- Safety
- The capacity to care for yourself and a partner
- A sense of commitment

WRITE AN AD FOR A LOVER WHO TOUCHES YOUR HEART AND SOUL

This can be a delightful opportunity for each of you to express your fantasies and dreams of all you wish for in an intimate partner. Give yourselves ten or fifteen minutes to compose this "personal ad," and be as sexy, soulful, inventive, funny, and specific as you know how. This is your chance to go over the top.

- Begin by writing, "WANTED . . . ," and then let your imagination run wild about what you want. (ISIS examples include: "a partner who taps into the deepest of my passions," or "who leaves no part of me untouched, from my eyelids to my toes," or "who cradles my fears and hopes and opens a door to cosmic love.") It's most important that you draw from your own wishes, but if you need ideas to get you started, look back through this book to see what ISIS women have said.
- Then write, "IN RETURN FOR WHICH . . . ," and be specific about what you would like to offer your ideal lover in the best of all possible worlds ("the most sensual massage you ever had," "a wild ride to the cosmos," or whatever moves you as being mutually delicious).

When you've finished writing these ads, read them aloud to each other. This presents a great opportunity for discussion (or direct action). Even if you don't have a partner, this can be a useful exercise to help free up your ideas about what an intimate sexual relationship could be for you. Sometimes I've asked workshop participants to write these ads for a lover. Then we've shuffled the answers and read them aloud in the group. This technique allows for a rich exchange of ideas and communication styles—and for anonymous feedback about what you want.

Here are some variations on this exercise you can also try:

- Write a "Letter to My Lover." You write this one directly to each other. Always begin with the positive, as it establishes the extent of your commitment and opens your partner to hearing you out. Write something you truly love about your partner, and follow with something you feel works really well for the two of you—whether or not it has to do directly with sex. The rest of the letter can focus on something you want your partner to understand about you—your wants, your needs, your fears, your wishes for contact, communication, and meaning. This is another opportunity to deepen your relationship through sharing feelings that may be difficult to bring up in the course of everyday life.

- Another variation is to address this letter to *yourself*. This brings home the idea that you are the most important sexual partner you'll ever have. And that true intimacy between partners begins with self-understanding and self-love.

REVERSE ROLES WITH YOUR PARTNER

ISIS values include the ability to tolerate a full range of feelings both in yourself and in your partner. This may sound easy, but in real life it can present difficulties, especially if you and your partner bring complicated histories into your relationship, or are overstressed with jobs, children, aging parents, and other necessaries of living. I've found that most partners truly want to understand each other deeply and fully, but they may get bogged down in conflicting feelings and endless details. This is a case where too much information can work against you.

A simple way for you and your partner to reach some profound mutual understanding is for the two of you to reverse roles for a short period of time. Take on each other's names and literally be each other—switch those bathroom towels marked His and Hers (or Hers and Hers if you're both women).

- Reverse roles for one hour. Do his chores, sit in her chair, watch his ballgame, express her attitudes, speak in his tone of voice, use her gestures, and so on. At the end of an hour discuss how it feels to inhabit each other's lives. What insights does this offer you about cooperation and empathy, and even sexual desire? What feelings does it raise? Talk about how you can use these insights and feelings to enhance your intimate relationship—as well as your relationships with others in your lives.

- To intensify this role reversal, make love *as each other*. That's right, switch—from your come-ons to your orgasmic patterns. This means not only playing out each other's sexual responses and routines but literally embodying each other as best you can. How does this expand your lovemaking repertoire? Does it make you more aware of each other? Does it help you ask for what you want? Perhaps it makes you giggle. (Laughing together is another way ISIS respondents say they deepen their sexual relationships.) Perhaps it feels painful—an opportunity to stop and discuss what isn't working.

WALK THE ISIS WHEEL WITH YOUR PARTNER

Adapt any of the exercises outlined in the previous chapter on walking the ISIS Wheel. Share your experiences with your partner, letting them take you both wherever you need to go. Some suggestions for adapting the ISIS Wheel to your partner relationship include:

- Trace the ISIS Wheel together and tell each other your feelings as you enter each path—physical, emotional, mental, and spiritual. This may launch an important discussion about the nature of your sexual relationship and what it means to you. Remember that ISIS respondents say sharing deep feelings is one of the major ways to bring spirituality into their sexual unions.

- Map an ISIS Wheel on your living room rug, put on your favorite music, and dance together all around the perimeter and through the paths, expressing your feelings as eloquently as you can through movement and body language—without words. This ISIS dance can intensify sexual intimacy, especially for couples who have difficulty talking about feelings.

- Re-create the ISIS Wheel in your bed and make love in the Center. You can position yourself along the various paths to indicate how you are responding, what you want, and where you'd like your partner to come with you. Try making love without a goal of intercourse or a goal of orgasm and notice if this changes the energy between you—and how you feel about the changes.

CHAPTER FOURTEEN

YOUR CHAKRAS, YOUR SELF

HAVE YOU EVER felt your body glow when you were making love? Or felt sparks—as if you were about to burst into flame? It's not all in your imagination. You were probably feeling energy radiating from your chakras—the powerful energy centers that exist throughout your body. Being aware of your chakras can help you understand your ISIS journey from an energetic point of view. This awareness can also extend your ISIS language by introducing you to a tradition of thought that honors the idea that sex can be a path to the soul.

Although the word "chakra" may sound New Agey, there's nothing new about it. The study of chakras is part of a serious and venerable yogic tradition dating back to fourth-century India. The chakra system is vast, but most diagrams of it include only seven major centers that correspond to nerves, glands, and vital organs. The three lower chakras are associated with how you relate to the physical world (and with your physical ISIS path). The four higher chakras are associated with emotional, mental, and spiritual issues (and with your other ISIS paths).

Chakra energy is believed to spin in circular patterns—*chakra* is the Sanskrit word for "wheel." Each chakra radiates out to the colorful energy field (or aura) that surrounds your body and links you with the world. When your energy is balanced, your chakras spin in harmony, your aura is bright and expansive, you feel healthy and optimistic. When your energy

MEANINGS, COLORS, AND SOUNDS USUALLY ASSOCIATED WITH CHAKRAS

CHAKRA LEVEL	MEANING	COLOR	SOUND
7, top of head, crown	Bliss, connection with universal energy, "I know"	Violet, white	*Nnng* (as in *sing*)
6, brow, third eye	Imagination, intuition, psychic "second sight," connection with archetypal patterns, "I see"	Indigo, amethyst	*Mmmm*
5, throat	Communication, creativity, expressiveness, "I reach out"	Blue	*Eeee*
4, heart	Love, self-acceptance, empathy, peace, community, "I love"	Pink, green	*Ahhh*
3, solar plexus	Power, will, ego, focus on self, rational thinking, "I deserve"	Yellow	*Awww*
2, sacrum	Emotional feelings, sexuality, desire, "I want"	Orange	*Oooh*
1, base of spine, perineum	Support, grounding, physical sensations, "I am"	Red	*Ohhh*

This table is based on information drawn from Barbara Brennan's Hands of Light *(Bantam, 1988), Rosalyn Bruyere's* Wheels of Light *(Fireside, 1994), and Anodea Judith's* Wheels of Life *(Llewellyn, 1999).*

is blocked, your chakras are sluggish, your aura is dull and constricted, and you feel sick and generally grumpy. There are countless variations between these two poles, of course. The point is (in this philosophy): You *are* your chakras. So it's important for you to know they exist, and how they affect you.

You may not be able to see all the colors of your aura, but you can sense your chakras once you know where they are and what they do. The best news is that you can learn to balance your chakra energies to enhance your health—and sexual health. By the end of this chapter you'll know how to give yourself regular chakra tune-ups—and how to attune your chakra energies with your partner's.

Some ISIS women describe their sexual experience in terms of chakras and auras. A Florida homemaker writes of color and light, and offers us an interesting insight into how sexual energy connects with spiritual energy:

> When we're making love, different colors escape from our auras—pink, blue, white, then when it gets really passionate the color turns deep purple. It is as if the auras from our souls join in spiritual union.

If you look on the chart above, you can see that the colors of the energy fields she mentions (pink, blue, purple, and white) match the colors of the four upper chakras—heart, throat, third eye, and crown. These are the "spiritual" chakras. Her experience is centered here, as distinct from her lower, or more "physical," chakras.

What I especially love about her description is that the spiritual chakras she alludes to directly correspond to the brain research findings detailed in chapter 11. Sophisticated imaging techniques now reveal that the temporal lobe, or "spiritual" center of the brain, can light up during physical arousal and orgasm. Women have been saying this in one form or another since time immemorial, but science hasn't been able to prove it until very recently. So this homemaker's description of connecting sex and spirit effectively spans two belief systems at once: the mystical and the scientific. In her words, the experience was "all-encompassing."

When your ISIS journey reaches the Center, all your paths—and all your chakras—are fully connected. The energy of that connection can create some mighty fine sensations, according to a therapist from Montana. In describing how her second chakra (sexuality) connects with her sixth chakra (intuition), she says it explicitly: "It feels as if the clitoris must be related to the third eye."

> When I have a strong orgasm, my body dissolves into light and I sense an opening in the third-eye area—an opening into unconditional love and/or a feeling of oneness with all. All fears and worries are forgotten. In fact it seems that when I am having frequent and full lovemaking, I rarely experience stress and overwhelming worries and fears. *It has the strength of prayer—it is a body prayer to love.*

What she's describing here is the movement of kundalini energy. The word "kundalini" comes from the Sanskrit *kunda,* which literally means "a lock of the beloved's hair." In energetic terms kundalini means creative potential. According to legend, this energy lies coiled like a serpent in the first chakra at the base of the spine. When the "energy serpent" is awakened, it uncoils upward through all the chakras and rises to activate the third eye and crown. In essence, this is an ISIS journey that connects the earthy roots of sexual desire with the sacred, loving, universal mind. It carries with it great strength, including the strength of prayer.

An author and producer from Canada writes about another aspect of ISIS chakra energy: the power to transform. She writes of her "soul-destroying" marriage to a man who refused to stand up for her in the face of his abusive grown children—a connubial hell, where communication had "crumbled into belittling snubs and angry retorts." For her the ISIS connection took the form of an orgasmic merging at what she calls the "soul level."

> One night as we lay in bed, gloomy in the blackness, I listened as he finally settled into sleep. I was lying there, hurting and questioning, when what I'm convinced is his soul—a blue light—lifted itself from his body, moved over to me, and somehow melted into my body. Every single inch of me was stroked by a body-length cellular orgasm. I will never

forget this moment. I hold it as the hope for reconciliation. No matter what he says, some part of him knows better.

Again, note the color, and look at the chakra chart above. A blue light moved from her husband's body to hers. This suggests that extraordinary throat chakra energy cleared their communication on a spiritual plane. It provided instant hope and meaning to a situation that she writes had been systematically killing her "cell by cell." And it provides us with a clear and colorful example of spiritual orgasm. Or as she phrased it, "orgasm without sex."

EXPLORING YOUR CHAKRA COLORS

Your chakra colors reflect the full spectrum of the rainbow, and they can be powerful balancers. You can work with chakra colors in any way that suits your lifestyle and imagination. You can visualize your chakra colors as you make love—one ISIS woman says she can orgasm up and down her chakras, so she can get a whole fabulous light show if she concentrates on the colors. You can reflect chakra colors in the clothing you wear (this is *way* beyond having your colors done by a department store color consultant). My dear friend Ruth Fishel, author of many meditation books, always wears some purple or violet to activate her intuition and imagination.

My personal favorite way of exploring my chakra colors is through a set of small polished gemstones, the kind you can pick up in any rock shop for a dollar or two. They're beautiful, they feel good in my hand, and they focus me on my chakra energies—which is helpful, because when I go overboard with my enthusiasms I easily lose balance.

Here are the stones I use:

Jasper—red, for the root chakra, grounding

Carnelian—orange, for the pelvic chakra, sexual energy

Citrine—yellow, for the solar plexus, power

Turquoise and rose quartz—green and pink, for the heart chakra, love

Lapis—blue, for the throat chakra, communication and creativity

Amethyst—purple, for the third eye, understanding and clairvoyance

Quartz crystal—clear, for the crown chakra, universal light

I play with these stones at my desk, or carry them in my pocket. Sometimes I line them up in the window and let the sun shine through them, and enjoy their beauty. I especially enjoy using them in the bathtub, and place them in different patterns in the water or on my body. Sometimes I hold them in my left hand and feel the energy that vibrates through them. Sometimes I meditate with them and listen to them talk to me. Stones have their own power, even their own language. They are known as the ancient wisdom keepers. They magnify our emotional and spiritual states—and they can help align you as you explore your ISIS paths.

Sounding Your Chakras

You can also explore your chakra energies by chanting the sounds associated with each chakra. (see the chart on page 141). This can be a powerful meditation to clear and balance yourself, and tune yourself for your ISIS journey. You can chant all of your chakras, you can concentrate on only one, or you can mix and match.

The point of sounding your chakras is to move your energy so that it uncoils up your body from the base of your spine to the top of your head, so that's how I it spell it out below. If this seems too hierarchical for you, feel free to play around with the sequence. Sounding your chakras might seem strange at first. But even if you feel self-conscious, think about giving it a try. Using your voice this way is like giving yourself a massage from the inside. Be prepared to feel relaxed, energized, and attuned—to your self, and to the universe.

There are numerous CDs that will help you sound the chakras—I particularly like Layne Redmond's *Chanting the Chakras*. If you're chanting on your own without a CD to accompany you, pitch your voice as low as you comfortably can for the first chakra, and pitch it higher with each successive chakra as you move up to your crown.

You can sit or stand or move your body as you sound your chakras. The point is to be comfortable.

1. Start at your *root chakra* with the sound *"ohhhh."* Feel your voice vibrate into the base of your spine. Feel yourself firmly connected to the ground. Chant until you feel rooted deeply in the earth. Chant "I am," and feel yourself embody the statement.

2. Sound your *second chakra* slightly higher with *"ooooh"* This is the chakra associated with the physical energy of sex. Feel your voice vibrate into your uterus, vagina, and clitoris. Put your hands on your belly just below your belly button. Move your pelvis and chant until you feel the roots of your sexual desire. Chant "I want," and feel yourself embody the statement.

3. Sound your *third chakra* with *"awwww."* Put your hands on your solar plexus. Feel your will. Feel your power pour up from your roots through to your chest and shoulders. Chant "I deserve," and fully feel your worthiness.

4. Sound your *heart chakra* with *"ahhhh."* Put your hands on your heart. Chant until you feel love surrounding you—pouring into you, pouring out from you. Chant "I love," and feel your heart open up and fill with acceptance.

5. Sound your *throat chakra* with *"eeeee."* With your fingers, pull the sound from your throat as if you were pulling taffy and sending its sweetness out into the world. Chant until you feel you are being fully heard. Chant "I communicate," and feel the resonance of your voice.

6. Sound your *third eye* with *"mmmmm"*—or use the universal sound *"om."* With your fingertips on your third eye—your brow—let yourself see as far as you can into the mysteries of the universe. Chant "I see," "I envision," "I understand," and welcome what comes to you.

7. Sound your *crown chakra* with *"nnnng"* (pronounced like "sing"), the sound of a bell. Hold your arms out and your hands up. Visualize your crown opening and light pouring in from the universe. My shamanic teacher uses an image I love: "Open your crown and let the sacred hummingbird drink the nectar there." Whatever image you use, this is the moment to visualize yourself opening to the universal mind and letting

all light and wisdom flow through you. Chant "I know," and fill with light from the universal mind.

After you've chanted your chakras, let the cumulative energy envelop you. Take time to notice how you feel—body, mind, heart, and soul. Feel—or imagine—your chakras spinning in harmony. Move your body, or rest, as spirit dictates. And know beyond the shadow of a doubt that your sexual energy is connected to all your other energies.

Sounding Your Chakras
with a Partner

You can also sound your chakras with your partner. This is an opportunity to make contact with each other through your voices, your hands, and your whole bodies. Chanting your heart chakras, is a wonderful opportunity for a heart-to-heart connection. Place your right hands on each other's hearts. Place your left hands over your own hearts as you chant *"ahhhh"* and look into each other's eyes.

In the process you can determine which of your chakra energies are matching. For instance, if you're both strong in heart energy (fourth chakra) or sexual energy (second chakra), your lovemaking will probably be very much in sync. But if your heart chakra is very strong and your partner is beaming out energy from the chakras associated with sex and will—your lovemaking could miss an essential connection. In effect, you'd be saying "I love" while your partner would be saying "I want" and "I deserve." As you sound your chakras together, imagine reaching out to give your partner some of your heart energy at the same time that you receive some sex—and will energy from your partner in return.

Sounding your chakras is a way to understand your sexual response as energy rather than as performance or an expression of gender or sexual orientation. It is also a natural place from which to move into Tantric sexual exercises in the next chapter.

CHAPTER FIFTEEN

TANTRA

Weaving New Sexual Possibilities

IN RECENT YEARS there has been an explosion of interest in Tantric sex. If you type the word "Tantra" into a Google search, you'll find nearly half a million websites, and a host of different avenues to explore, from "sacred loving" to "horny matches." There's even a site that proclaims, "Christian Sex Expert Shows Husbands How to Make Love for Hours."

Dozens of ISIS women name Tantra as the practice that helped move them beyond the performance model of sex. You don't have to know all the fine points of Tantra in order to experience fulfilling and meaningful sex, but some of the basic teachings and practices may enrich your ISIS journey. At the very least, it may help you to know that there's an established religious tradition that confirms the idea that sex can be much more than "wham-bam-thank-you-ma'am"—that physical sex can be deeply connected with our highest spiritual values.

Tantra originated in the context of ancient Hinduism and Tibetan Buddhism. Authentic Tantra comprises a complex and vast set of spiritual teachings that are traditionally given only to those who have undergone years of spiritual practice and study. In the 1970s Tantra was popularized in the Western world by controversial sex guru Bhagwan Sri Rajneesh (Osho), and in the 1980s by author and teacher Margo Anand—two of her best-selling books are *The Art of Sexual Ecstasy* and *The Art of Sexual Magic*.

One of the basic Tantric teachings is that the wide and tactile universe was conceived through sex—through the union of sacred beings—not through a collision of atoms or the sudden command of God. Another basic teaching is that the human body and the cosmos are mirror images of one another. That is, each of us carries the patterns of the entire universe in our DNA, so our most profound sexual experiences naturally embody the mysteries of the cosmos. (If you wonder about the hard science of all this, read Jeremy Narby's curious book, *The Cosmic Serpent*. He's an anthropologist and chemist who's gifted at explaining spiritual belief systems in scientific language.) In the Tantric view, our earthly sexual unions are sacred. The deities are our mentors and also our mirrors—in the language of the ancient alchemists, "As above, so below."

Another Tantric teaching is about uniting the great dualities—sex and spirit, human and divine—the kinds of opposites mentioned at the beginning of this book. "Tantra" comes from the Sanskrit word for weaving, and ISIS women describe Tantra as connecting different strands of their sexuality. A forty-six-year-old hospital chaplain from Denver writes of using Tantric practices to help "integrate the male and female within." A forty-seven-year-old music therapist from Fort Collins, Colorado, says Tantra helps her "make sense of her whole life."

The acceptance that the body is a gift to be appreciated, just like nature's other gifts, opens the gateway to living life in the fullness of its joys and sorrows. Like light and shadow, one enhances the other.

These and other teachings of Tantra hold some powerful wisdom for women today. They can help us heal the sexual wounds that so many of us carry in our bodies, minds, and spirits—guilt, shame, and lack of confidence. And Tantric practices can be a blessing for women with physical disabilities, as they take the sexual focus off physical athleticism and place it in your heart and soul—your ability to move energy.

In Tantric practice you and your partner make love not only with your bodies and your egos. You also make love as deities—to honor the god and goddess within yourselves. Your goal is transcendence and enlightenment. According to feminist scholar Miranda Shaw, Tantra can move you to a "higher octave" of sexual autonomy, agency, affirmation, and liberation—that is, deep soul connections with your partner, and also with *you*. As one ISIS woman says, "I understand others in a way I never did before, and the world seems a far less lonely place . . . it brings me home to myself."

The Ritual Practices

The ancient texts on Tantric sex elaborated countless rules for courting, kissing, sexual play, intercourse, and using aphrodisiacs (an early version of today's performance-enhancing drugs). These rules were universally addressed to heterosexual couples, and mostly to the men—who were actually taught to drain female energy from their partners to speed their own journey to enlightenment. I have come to view this as a sanctified form of sexual vampirism, and very different from the highest spiritual principles of Buddhist and Hindu thought. But thanks to the women's movement and the march of time, today's Tantric techniques are usually based on sharing energies, and generating plenty for everyone—women as well as men, and gay and lesbian partners, too.

As it's most often practiced in the West today, Tantric sex involves some basic lovemaking rituals to help couples move from physical sensation to higher consciousness. These range from eye contact to appreciation and worship. All are aimed to inspire the rising of energy coiled in the pelvis (that's the kundalini serpent we met in the chapter on chakras).

The practices listed below are ones ISIS women mention most often. But there are hundreds of Tantric techniques, chants, and yoga postures. A wealth of information is available on the Internet, in books, and on videos and DVDs. I invite you to explore all of the above along with the suggested readings at the back of this book. My personal favorites are the books by Miranda Shaw and Tsultrim Allione, because they shed such clear light on Tantra as an empowering practice for women.

MEDITATION

Tantric meditation typically begins with an invocation of deities—often highly erotic love songs to the sacred couple, Shakti and Shiva. Here sexual intention merges with religious worship. The meditation itself can become a vital expression of sexual energy as well as a preliminary to physical sex. ISIS women say it can be mind-altering, time-altering, spirit-invoking, and so satisfying to the internal senses that there may be no urgency for physical sensation. The goal of Tantric meditation is perfect awareness and freedom of both body and spirit. Result: divine ecstasy—and a powerful way to align your ISIS consciousness with a practice that already has a proven history.

You don't have to adhere to exact religious traditions in order to experience some of the benefits of Tantra—although there are workshops all over the country where you can learn techniques of Tantric meditation. You can simply follow your breath and quiet your mind as a preliminary to physical lovemaking, as many ISIS women do. "Opening our hearts to God and each other," says one woman. "Overcoming the barriers of fear so we can just be one in the moment," says another. A fifty-six-year-old physical therapist from Putney, Vermont, writes that she listens to different parts of herself to learn where she is in a sexual situation. "I literally 'check in.' For me it is necessary to experience that balance in order to be sexual with another." She also describes what she calls "conscious synchronicity" in a heart and body meditation with a beloved partner:

> Often we would just sit in front of each other and allow the energy to flow into sex slowly and with intention on full heart and full body. Our minds were at ease in that time because we would bring our attention to each other and let other preoccupations drift away.

GAZING

Gazing is one of the classic Tantric techniques for expanding the capacity for pleasure. An ISIS woman from Tucson is a Tantra teacher who describes herself as "spirit in a fifty-year-old body." She writes of finding "windows to the universe" through the ritual practice of gazing—that is, allowing your sexual energy to express itself through your eyes rather than the usual channels of hands, lips, and genitals. "With every sexual partner," she says, "there were flashes of universes beyond the physical act of joining." She describes a multidimensional sexual journey she initiated by gazing.

> I wanted to be fully aware of the sexual experiences we were having and kept my eyes open more than usual. At one point during intercourse, he opened his eyes also. As our eyes met, I felt that we were seeing our souls and I could see and feel eternity.

Tantric gazing can take various forms. It can mean emptying your mind, softening your focus, and looking into the middle distance. For Tantra aficionados it can mean concentrating on a *yantra*, a diagram of the sexual energy created by the union of the cosmic couple, of Shakti and Shiva.

For most ISIS women it means gazing at your partner and into your partner. This is more than appreciating a glossy body or pretty face. It means looking intently into the heart of your beloved, looking into the eyes of your beloved, and like the teacher above, looking through your beloved's eyes into the eyes of the universe. This kind of gazing can be a most intimate act. It contains and channels your sexual energy and releases it into pure spirit. Try gazing deeply into your own heart as well—where your desires meet your beliefs and truths.

APPRECIATING THE GENITALS

In Tantric terminology, appreciating the genitals is called *yoni and lingam puja*. ("Yoni" means vulva. "Lingam" means penis. "Puja" means worship.) Worshipping the genitals is powerful and reverent, like worshipping a diety. The form of this worship ranges from gazing, to gentle caressing, to massaging the "sacred spot" (otherwise known as your G spot) inside the front wall of your vagina. (If you don't know how to find your G spot or what it can do for you, you can learn all about it in the newly reissued 1980s best seller, *The G Spot*.) Skillful, loving G-spot massage feels wonderful for some women, and it can ultimately stimulate ejaculation as well as orgasm, which is a whole other story you can read about in that book.

Yoni and lingam puja stands in strong contrast to our culture's attitudes toward the genitals. On the one hand we see our genitals as shameful or embarrassing; on the other we seem obsessed with what size they are, how juicy they are, and how well they perform. (One of today's onslaught of spam e-mails proclaims, "Gain Up to Three Inches in Length—No Surgery, No Side Effects!") ISIS women say a Tantric flow of appreciation for each other's genitals opens them to the flow of universal love.

One of my teachers at the Institute for Advanced Study of Human Sexuality was Kenneth Ray Stubbs, who is the author of many books on sacred sex. Even before Tantra became popular in this country, he was teaching a "Secret Garden" massage that reverently connects the breasts, vulva, and penis, connecting them with the rest of the body. He maintains that leaving out your genitals is nothing more than a "doughnut" massage—about as nourishing as junk food, and a hefty just-say-no message about sexual pleasure. His illustrated book, *The Essential Tantra*, is a complete guide to sensitive, sensual, sexual massage that brilliantly includes all of you.

TANTRIC ORGASM

In the performance model of sex, the goal is to climax with orgasm, an explosion of physical energy. Not so in Tantra, where you linger in the process of gazing, worship, and attention to your sacred partner. Vigorous thrusting is a no-no for the most part. Both men and women learn techniques to diffuse and delay orgasm and ejaculation. The Tantric ideal is to maintain a kind of flow—a state of shared physical and spiritual bliss that doesn't require an erect penis or even a lubricated vagina, and that can last "well, in some sense, forever," says one ISIS woman.

A forty-four-year-old chiropractor from Palm Springs, California, speaks of experiencing a "chakra wave" with her partner: "Tremendous energy was streaming through my third, fourth, and fifth chakras to my third eye and crown. Then light, bliss, and ecstasy!" If you consult the chakra chart in chapter 14, you san see that the sexual energy she describes was clearly not confined to her genitals. It moved through her solar plexus, her heart, and her throat to her upper chakras, which are associated with vision, bliss, and connection with the divine union. The orgasm she's describing is an opening to transpersonal, universal consciousness. In Tantric terms, this is the blooming of the "thousandpetaled lotus."

Many ISIS women describe similar experiences even though they've never heard of Tantra. They speak of "heart orgasms," "soul orgasms," "love orgasms." They speak of orgasms that require no physical touch—sponta-neous orgasms, or "thinking off"—you met these orgasms in chapter 7, on beliefs and messages. Many women say their orgasms are born from the energy of their soul-mate relationships. An eighteen-year-old from Wilm-ington, North Carolina, writes, "When I unite with another person sexu-ally, it is an expression of two divine energies channeling through two bodies to create the highest form of balance and consciousness."

It's no wonder that author Margo Anand calls Tantra "high sex." Tantra can lead us to the highest vibrations of our sexual and spiritual energies. There are practitioners who spend a lifetime learning its nuances—maybe several lifetimes if you listen to some adepts and gurus. A sixty-three-year-old therapist, who writes that she's studied Tantra since the 1970s, expresses the connection between Tantric teachings and the ISIS Wheel. Both embody a journey from physical delight to spiritual wisdom, and some-times from darkness and fear into the realm of universal love. "I believe I have been richly blessed to have explored the shadow side of sexuality as well as the light, and to have come through that time with wisdom and understanding."

CHAPTER SIXTEEN

CREATING SEXUAL CEREMONY

INCORPORATING SOME ELEMENTS of ceremony into sex can be a powerful way to enrich your ISIS experience. Ritual and ceremony aren't for everybody, of course. And some women feel decidedly uncomfortable about the idea of bringing anything that seems remotely like religion into their bedrooms. Still others feel that having to create sexual ceremony actually acts as a barrier to ISIS— adding more prep work and another sexual goal to achieve, when what they really want to do is keep it simple.

But if the idea of ceremonial and ritual elements in lovemaking feels inspiring to you, read on. Sexual ceremony can provide a degree of attention and awareness that deepens sexual experiences and helps make them transformative. It's guaranteed to take sex beyond the performance model—out of the realm of routine intercourse and into something memorable, perhaps into the very center of the ISIS Wheel. Read how a forty-seven-year-old musician from Austin, Texas, describes an elaborate process of invocation, cleansing, music, and prayers as part of the lovemaking ritual with her husband.

We stated our intention that it be a rich experience of our love as a gift to and from God. We called in our guides and the master teachers. We cleansed the energy in the house with incense and chanting. Then we bathed and got into silk clothes for dancing. We then said a long prayer and sang thanks for our many blessings. Then we went into the sound room—an acoustic dream room, 40 feet by 25 feet, designed for live music—and drummed and danced and sang and laughed and laughed and felt deliriously happy to be alive. We kissed, we sang, we told each other why we appreciate each other, we caressed, we danced, we breathed together—the whole experience lasted many, many hours.

ISIS women write of many other ways it's possible to create sexual ceremony—you don't have to have a sound studio or practice a certain religion. There are also books that offer abundant details—I especially recommend Margo Anand's *The Art of Sexual Ecstasy*, Linda Savage's *Reclaiming Goddess Sexuality*, Ray Stubbs's *Essential Tantra*, and Jenny Wade's *Transcendent Sex*. All are in the suggested readings.

Here is a basic recipe for creating powerful sexual ceremony. Like all recipes, the flavor improves as you add your own individual touches, which may change each time you practice.

SETTING THE STAGE

However informal your ceremony might be, it's crucial that you set the stage. Your stage doesn't have to be grand, but you do need to differentiate it from your everyday stomping grounds. Clean and clear the space where you're going to hold your sexual ceremony. This might include dusting, vacuuming, neatening, and putting fresh sheets on your bed. Create privacy by making sure you won't be interrupted by telephone, children, or visitors. If your ceremony is to be outdoors, make sure the space is comfortable, protected, free of debris—and free of neighbors.

PREPARING YOURSELF

It's important to enter into your ceremony with an open heart so that you can clarify your intentions and feelings. What do you want to do? What do you want the outcome to be? Will your ceremony include a partner or is it for yourself alone? Will your ceremony include physical sex? If not, you can also ceremonially prepare yourself for sexual fantasy and erotic meditation.

Once you're clear on these questions, you (and your partner, if a partner is involved) need to clear yourselves. You can clear away the tensions of the day by bathing or showering. You can pamper your body with lotions or oils. You can brush your skin and hair with your hands, flowers, or feathers. You can purify your energy by "smudging" yourself with smoke from herbs, such as cedar and white sage. To do this, you burn a few dried herbs in a flameproof container, then with your hands or a feather you brush the smoke slowly over each of your chakras (see the chakra chart in chapter 14).

Smudging yourself may sound somewhat "woo-woo" if you've never experienced it. But this method of purification has been practiced for centuries in native ceremonies. It's a preamble to healing as well as to worship. Adrienne Borden, a physician at the East West College of Natural Medicine in Sarasota, Florida, writes that she was taught to intuit the dark spots in a person's energy field and to brush the smoke into those spots to "close up" the holes and promote healing.

CREATING SACRED SPACE

Once you've set the stage and prepared yourself, you're ready to create the actual space in which your sexual ceremony will take place—whether it's in your bed, or living room, or a tent outdoors. Some women feel it's important to create a special altar. This can be as simple as lighting a candle by your bedside. Or it can be an elaborate arrangement of stones, feathers, shells, flowers, photos—whatever is meaningful and sacred to you. Some women imagine their bed as a kind of altar to Eros, or to the goddess of love.

If you sense any negativity in your sacred space, take charge immediately and command it to leave. You can do this quite simply by clapping your hands. If the negativity feels heavy, shout! Tell it to begone! Clap and shout until you feel the energy lighten up. I've counseled some couples to clear the way for lovemaking by becoming Energy Bouncers, literally throwing the memory of a disapproving or abusive parent out of the bedroom.

Once you've exorcised any heaviness, there are various ways to open the energy in your sacred sexual space. Smudging the space with sacred smoke is part of the opening ritual in spiritual traditions the world over, from ancient earth religions to the Roman Catholic Church. You can smudge your space in the same spirit you smudged yourself. Ringing bells is another technique used in many traditions—you can hear the vibrations literally clear the air. You can sing or chant words to bring lightness back to the space. I like to play a cedar flute because its voice opens both my throat and my heart at the same time. The important thing is to be inventive and true to yourself. Listen closely to what the situation calls for and then do what you're most moved to do.

OFFERING GIFTS

It's traditional to bring gifts to a ceremonial space as offerings to the divine forces you want to invoke. Flowers are a fine ISIS offering for both the romantic and spiritual aspects of your ritual. Ceremonial offerings can also include other gifts of the earth, such as cornmeal, tobacco, or wine—fruits of the vine. Andean *curanderas* (women healers) believe that the helping spirits are especially partial to sweet smells and tastes, so they load their altars with incense, carnations, and chocolate. Offer whatever feels right to you—you can include songs, prayers, poems, meditations, or dance. Repeat your focused intentions. You can use your breath to blow your intentions and your name into the center of the space—as an offering of yourself.

CALLING IN HELPFUL ENERGIES

You can call in the natural world: the earth, the sky, and the four cardinal directions—south, west, east, and north. You can invoke the elements of air, fire, earth, and water. You can call in the emotional energies you want present at your ceremony, such as love, passion, and compassion. You can name helpful deities—Isis, Mary, Shekhinah, Quan Yin, and Pachamama are all powerful nurturing goddesses from very different cultures (Egyptian, Christian, Hebrew, Chinese, and Andean). Different spiritual traditions assign different meanings to these directions, elements, and deities, and you might add some special meanings of your own. If you belong to a Judeo-Christian religion, it may help you to know that all of our mainstream religions developed out of ancient earth-centered practices and that vestiges of these practices (such as invoking the deity) remain in our various liturgies today. An Internet search is an easy way to find an overview of various traditions, from Tibetan Buddhism to Wiccan communities.

You have a wide choice of ways you can call in all these helpful energies. Some women use ritual chants or hymns that they take from traditions they know. Some use percussion instruments—rattles and drums, gongs, and cymbals. Some use wind instruments—flutes, trumpets, conch shells, didgeridoos. Some use dance and gestures along with sound. Some simply use intention—the power of your heart and mind. Use whatever methods you feel can most powerfully call in what, and whom, you want to be present at your ISIS ceremony.

If you've never called in the spirits before, you may feel a bit shy about speaking out loud to the unseen world. I felt quite tongue-tied when I began, but soon learned that it works. If you call, they listen. It was a question of letting go of my ego and understanding that this wasn't a speaking engagement I was being judged on. This was a way of establishing a personal intimate relationship with the divine. In other words, prayer.

THE CORE OF YOUR CEREMONY

Once you've set the stage, you're ready to create the core of your ceremony. This can take any form you choose. You can step into the center of the ISIS Wheel with your partner—as outlined in chapter 13. You can explore any aspect of your sexuality with or without a partner. You can practice Tantric gazing. Or you can just make something up as you go along. Your preparations may have increased your level of anticipation and desire. Allow the energy you've already created to begin to move in you—whether this becomes deep meditation or external body movement. Breathe deeply into any movement, sound, or images. Be aware of the motion in every chakra. Feel the exchange of energy between you and your environment. Feel the exchange of energy between you and your partner. Let yourself go into orgasmic release if that is what occurs naturally without becoming the ultimate goal.

Here, of course, resides the center of your ceremony. This may be short and sweet, or it may continue on all night, as it did for the musician quoted at the opening of this chapter. The ISIS stories throughout this book are testimony to the range and variety of experiences you might enjoy along the way.

CLOSING THE CIRCLE

When your ceremony is complete, it's supremely important that you close the space. Think of all the energies and beings you called in to help you. You opened a portal for them—and for other energies too. It's kind of like giving an open house at holiday time. People come and bring their friends. It's wonderful to have everyone over, but at some point you're ready for them to go home and for you to reclaim your space. Imagine what might occur if you kept that invitation open forever. You don't know who might wander in. So keep things neat. Close up the space when you're ready to move on.

There are many ways to do this. I like to begin by offering gratitude—appreciation and praise. Thank your partner and any others who've been part of the ceremony. Thank yourself for your openness in engaging in this process. Thank the space. Thank the spirits and energies who have been present. Thank the directions and the elements. Release them, and invite them to come back when you call on them again.

You can embellish these thank-yous with words, movement, chants, and instruments. Or you can close the circle silently. It's really your intention that counts. My shamanic teacher, Oscar, has a method of closing his ceremonial circles that is both elegant and effective. I offer my adaptation of it here, and invite you to further adapt it to fit your own situation.

OSCAR'S CLOSING

When you're ready, face the center of your ceremonial space (or you can face each other if your partner has been part of the ceremony).

Take a full breath in and hold it. With your left hand, scoop up all the good feelings that have been created. Place your left hand over your heart.

Hold your breath for a count of three, drinking in all the good feelings.

Aim the palm of your right hand to the center of the space (or place it on your partner's heart).

Now blow all those good feelings back into the center of the space (or into your partner's heart chakra). This is the spirit of sacred reciprocity, giving back what you have received.

Take another deep breath and hold it. Place your right hand over your left—on your own heart. On a count of three blow the good feelings toward the heavens—to distribute them freely into the universe—again in a spirit of sacred reciprocity.

Finally, hold your arms in front of you at shoulder height, and on a count of three clap your hands together to seal the ceremony. It is done.

Extinguish any candles or incense, and return the space to resume its function in your daily life.

CHAPTER SEVENTEEN

ELF AND WAIF

Updating Your Sexual History—
With Love

ALMOST ALL OF US have some degree of vulnerability around our sexual relationships. It may be anxiety, fear, anger, avoidance, or simply shyness. These can be difficult issues to explore. First of all, who wants to delve into old negative yuck? But negative yuck has a way of bubbling up from the past when you least expect it. And it can sabotage your adult sexual relationships. This is especially true if it's attached to sexual trauma or abuse or deeply embedded messages that undermine your right to pleasure. Some women feel they'll never be totally yuck-free.

Here is an interactive meditation to help you update your sexual history—with love. You're going to call on the wisdom of your inner children: your "Elf," who carries the positive energy of your past, and your "Waif," who carries the negativity.

To receive full measure from this exercise, give yourself plenty of time—and stay as open as you can while your journey unfolds. Prepare yourself as you might for a sexual encounter—perhaps with a soothing bath or some light exercise. Clear your mind and your space as you might for a spiritual practice. Make sure there'll be no interruptions. You can light candles, put on meditative music—whatever helps you focus.

Invoking Your Elf and Waif
An Interactive Meditation

Close your eyes and be aware of your breathing. Let the rhythm of your breathing bring you to the perimeter of the ISIS Wheel—the place where sexuality intersects with your life. As you stand here in the present, know that the paths of the ISIS Wheel lead far into your future and way back into your earliest memory. Notice how you feel standing at this midpoint in your life. And breathe—in and out.

In your imagination, walk around the ISIS Wheel and be aware of a path opening to you. This is your entry point to your journey through your past experience. Is the path that opens before you physical, emotional, mental, or spiritual? Or have you moved right into the Center? Become instantly aware. Don't try to choose a more "perfect" way. This path has chosen you. Know that where you are connects with all of the other ISIS paths. And that you may change paths at any point during your journey. Notice what this path looks like and how it feels under your feet. What colors, textures, and other sensations are you aware of as you begin to walk this path in your imagination? And remember to breathe.

Allow your breath to lead you back into your past. On this path, begin to walk your way back through all the years to before you were an adult. And past your adolescent years—until you reach your childhood. You come upon a little girl huddled in the dirt. Her eyes are your eyes, and they tug at your heart. You recognize her as your long-ago child of disappointment, trauma, and betrayed trust. I call her your inner Waif—but you may have another name for her.

Let the right name come as you breathe in and out.

Invite her to join you on your journey through your past. As you walk with her, ask her about herself. How old is she? What's happening in her life that makes her sad and scared? What are the sexual messages she's learned? Take her hand in yours as you walk. Be aware of how it feels to touch your inner Waif. And keep breathing.

Confide in her. Tell her you know she shows up during your sexual encounters in the present. You can tell when she's hiding under the bed. You know when she's getting between you and your partner. You know when she's feeling whiny or having a tantrum. Let her know now that you understand why she's acting like this. But also let her know that from now on you'd like your sexual encounters to be clearer and happier for you both. Breathe in rhythm with her now.

Ask her what she needs from you. As the adult, you need to know how you can help her feel safe when you're in a sexual situation now. Perhaps there's some information she can give you. Maybe she needs reassurance, some special kind of recognition or attention. Breathe together with her. Let her answer clearly. And listen closely to her answer. Notice where you feel her answer in your body. And breathe.

Tell her what you'd like from her. In fact, you may want her to get lost. But she can't, and you can't make her. She's a part of you. So tell her you need her cooperation. And tell her exactly how you'd like her to behave. Perhaps you'd like her to sit quietly in a corner and amuse herself while you get on with your adult sexual responses. Perhaps you wish you could borrow her soulfulness to bring with you on your sexual journey. Maybe you'd just like her to quit tugging on you. Whatever you want from her, let her know now.

Listen to her response. Really listen, and take it in until she feels you've heard her. Then you may need to negotiate with her so that each of you can feel safe and happy. Take time to do that now. And breathe.

When you're ready, notice that a second little girl has joined you. You can see at a glance that she's filled with joy. She's interested, alive, aware. She bounces over to you and says, "Hi!" She is your inner Elf. Being near her lifts your heart. Reflect this lightness in your breath. If you feel like making some sound, feel free to do that now.

Reach out to her with your other hand. Invite her to accompany you and your Waif on your journey. Notice how it feels to hold her hand. And to breathe with her.

Have the same conversation you just had with her sister Waif—and remember to breathe:

- Let her name come to you.
- How old is she?
- What's happening in her life?

- Confide in her about her presence on your sexual path.
- Ask how you can help make your sexual experiences safe and happy for her.
- Say what you want from her when you're in a sexual situation.
- Hear her responses clearly. And breathe.

Gather both Elf and Waif in your arms and breathe together. Introduce them to each other. Embrace them. Enjoy them. Take your time. They are the core of your inner family. And they are an important part of your sexual energy and spirit. They live in that place between your breathing in and breathing out. A place of transformation.

Let them hear that you'll find ways to protect and nurture them both. Assure them that they are part of your spirit—and that sexual expression is part of your spirit too. You're all in it together. Let yourself see your updated information about safe and happy lovemaking written out in your own handwriting. Or maybe in sky writing. Or in an e-mail attachment. Or a greeting card. However you receive this information, put it into an envelope and tuck it next to your heart.

Follow your breath back into the here-and-now. When you feel ready, open your eyes and notice your surroundings. Be aware that you've contacted an essential part of yourself and of your sexual energy—these beings who are embedded in your breath and imprinted in your heart and soul. Know that you can contact them again whenever you want. And that you can always look into your heart and open the envelope containing the updated information you need.

Once you've contacted your Elf and Waif (by whatever names you want to call them), it's important to talk about your journey. This gives witness to yourself and validates your experience. Also, talking out loud may offer insight and direction as you update your old messages about sex and love. This is deep and vulnerable material that lies at the core of your sexuality. Choose a person you know will understand—your partner or someone else you trust. Writing about your discoveries in your journal is another option if you can't immediately find the right person to talk with.

Feel free to adapt this meditation to fit your life. Maybe there are other voices that need to speak. Maybe your issue isn't abuse or negative messages. If not, choose an issue to explore where you feel you need an inner dialogue to update your sexual feelings. The point is to tune into a crucial transformational truth: You can change the present and the future by acknowledging the past and how it's affected you. And you can change the effects of the past by becoming more aware in the present.

CHAPTER EIGHTEEN

DESIDERATA

Your Rights to Intimacy
and Pleasure

IT'S IMPORTANT FOR YOU to know what your sexual rights are—no matter what your age or sexual orientation or physical ability. Some of us seem to know our rights instinctively and are able to set effective boundaries and ask for what we want. But many of us have never thought about our rights to intimacy and pleasure—or even imagined that we had such rights. When we're unaware, we're extra vulnerable to being taken advantage of by others, whether they intend to take advantage of us or not.

I originally devised the bill of rights below with Beverly Whipple when we were writing *Safe Encounters,* the first book to guide women how to say yes to pleasure and no to unsafe sex. Here, in the context of ISIS, I want to link it with your longings for heart and soul connection as well as for physical safety. The word "desiderata" means "the things you desire."

My Rights to Intimacy
and Pleasure

1. I have a right to my own body and all of its sensations, including pleasure and pain.
2. I have a right to think my own thoughts, whatever they may be.
3. I have a right to feel the full range of my emotions—excitement, joy and anger, sorrow and depression, love and fear—whether or not my feeling them is acceptable to others.
4. I have a right to acknowledge my memories, whether they are memories of delight or of abuse, and to base present relationship decisions on them.
5. I have a right to be—or not to be—a sexual person at all ages and stages of my life, and a right to choose how I define what I mean by sexuality.
6. I have a right to expect that my partner respect my body, thoughts, feelings, and general well-being, and a right to insist on respect, if necessary.
7. I have a right to ask for what I want.
8. I have a right to say no to any sexual encounter that feels unsatisfying or threatening—physically, emotionally, spiritually, or sexually.
9. I have a right to say yes to pleasure that is physically, emotionally, spiritually, and sexually safe.
10. I have a right to feel good about saying both yes and no.

I've often used this list with clients, college students, health professionals, and other groups. It's an effective and moving way to start discussions about what women really want—and don't want. I especially love bringing it into small groups, where women can read these rights around a circle. Each woman reads one, then passes the page on to the woman next to her. When there are more than ten women in the group, we keep passing the page until each woman has had a chance to declare at least one right. (When there are fewer than ten women, we pass the page around until all the rights are declared.)

It's important for us not only to know our rights but to say them out loud. Too many of us have never spoken up. When we do speak up in safety, we invariably feel validated. I can't tell you how many times I've heard: "That statement I just read—it must've been written just for me."

Here's a variation on this bill of rights that came to me in 1998 when my daughter and I were traveling in the Black Hills of South Dakota. In that lovely land sacred to the first Americans, it became clear to me that our rights to intimacy and pleasure are connected to timeless truths. The words below came through as guidance straight to my heart. I offer them here to you with proper attribution.

GUIDANCE FROM THE GODDESSES OF LOVE

1. Your body knows.
2. Trust what you see with your eyes closed.
3. You are protected.
4. Sense and spirit are tides in the same ocean.
5. Speak until you're sure you are heard.
6. If you remember it, it probably happened.
7. Memories make good compost. Be patient.
8. Reach for the ripest plum in the bowl.
9. You don't have to eat it.
10. Feeling good takes practice.

Maybe you have some items you'd like to add to the lists above. Or maybe you want to make your own list from scratch. Maybe you have specific desires that aren't included here. Or specific boundaries you need to mention.

I encourage you to be as creative as you wish. If writing isn't your thing, draw what you want, make a collage with magazine scraps, or act your wishes out with your body. What's really important here is that you think out the rights and truths and desires that are essential for you. Put them out where you can see them. Say them out loud. Discuss them with your friends. With your partner. Most of all, make certain that you know in your own heart exactly what they are.

CHAPTER NINETEEN

INVOKING YOUR KEEPER OF THE FLAME

IN THE FIRST PART of this book, I issued an invitation for you to take a quantum leap and begin thinking about your sexuality in a new, more complex way. I invited you into the ISIS Wheel of Sexual Experience—to follow your paths of body, mind, heart, and spirit to the magical places where they meet. Now, here's a further invitation. It's a call to invoke the "Keeper of the Flame" of your sexual energy. Communicating with this being can help you move beyond limiting performance definitions of sexual response. It can even move you beyond what you think you already know about your sexuality. Here I invite you to dive deep into your own imagination to meet your personal guide and teacher—a wise and wonderful mentor who awaits within you to help you discover all that sexual wholeness means for you.

If this sounds as if I'm asking you to leave the comfort of your judgments and prejudices about your sexuality, I am—but if you really don't want to give them up, you can always return to your old ways once the journey is over. It might encourage you to know that I've led hundreds of women on similar journeys, and I've learned that this experience can hold powerful medicine no matter what you bring to it.

At journey's end, many women have tales to tell—stories of going to far places in their imaginations, stories of change and transformation, and sometimes puckish humor. One of my personal favorites is from a psychiatrist colleague who came to a workshop feeling wildly conflicted about whether or not to become pregnant. Her Keeper of the Flame appeared to her as—guess what—a baby! The message was clear. It was time for her to activate the generative, nurturing part of her sexual being. A year to the day after she embarked on this inner journey, her son, Noah, was born. As far as I know, she's the only woman who's ever gotten pregnant from doing this exercise.

Other women received messages that spoke to other concerns in their lives. One whose husband had walked out years before received a radiant valentine, which said to her that she was finally ready for new love. A teacher from Connecticut who had been struggling with autoimmune problems said the gift she experienced was a sense of alchemical change—she felt her entire system turn from lead to gold. Although this gift was mystical and metaphorical, it encouraged her to trust that she was on the road to vibrant physical health, which happily turned out to be quite true.

But no story unfolded in as much detail as that of a forty-eight-year-old journalist who wrote me a wonderful letter three weeks after she'd experienced her journey. This is a woman who had entered the workshop feeling small and spent. She'd been through a contentious divorce. Her mother had recently died. Her goal for the weekend was to bridge what she saw as a yawning divide between her sexual nature and her spiritual nature. She wanted to stop feeling ashamed. She wanted to stop withdrawing. In her words, she wanted "to come out more as a sexy woman, a woman who wants to be seen in her fullness, who is not afraid that being sexual somehow diminishes or negates all the other aspects of her self-expression."

Her Keeper of the Flame appeared at once—"a naked, dancing, playful, pagan priestess. She fairly leaped and skipped ahead of me." Her Keeper led her to a Goddess of Sexual Wholeness—a huge and powerful figure who had the ability to nurture. She also had the ability to shape-shift—which is one of the unique qualities of spirit beings.

At first she looked like a Botticelli Venus and I thought, "No, she doesn't have to be blond and classically beautiful. She could look more like me." Then she shifted through all colors of skin and hair and was very big and imposing. And I realized I could crawl up inside her womb. When I did, it was a large space, very dark yet also comfortable and safe.

The deepest recesses of our imaginations have their ways of telling the truth even when our waking selves are distracting us with busy-ness and drama. For this ISIS woman, the images of Mother and Goddess of Sexual Wholeness merged—powerfully enough to override the just-say-no legacy from her biological mother, who had been deeply ashamed of sex. This was the instant of magic, when the dead weight in her system seemed to turn to gold—just as it had for the teacher with the autoimmune problem.

I felt what it was like to have a mother who was strong and powerful enough to really take care of me, to give me what I needed in a way my personal mother had not been fully able to do. And perhaps most important, since she was the Goddess of Sexual Wholeness, she was not ashamed and she could birth me without shame. I could come into my life without the burden of shame about my body and sexuality. The energy in my body continued to move with shaking and sobs as I felt the full impact of these images . . . [including] an image of being held against her breast and soothed.

The changes were immediate—and were reflected in her body. At the end of the journey, everyone in the room noticed that she'd grown straighter, even larger. Her face was smooth, her voice resonant and confident. We've been in touch over the years and these responses have withstood the test of time. She not only lived the journey in the moment, she's kept the spirit of the journey strong within her.

It feels like a touchstone I can return to when I come up against fear, doubt, and shame on my journey to fully claiming my sexuality. I am very grateful for this journey, for this experience. To have the chance to redeem the ideal of Mother as Virgin and replace it with the experience of Mother as wholly, holy sexual Goddess.

Journey to Your Keeper
of the Flame

You don't need to attend a special workshop to journey to your Keeper of the Flame. You can embark on this journey by yourself, or with a partner. Anyone can do it. It's not rocket science. This kind of imaginative journey requires no special esoteric skills. You can even sleep through it and come away with something meaningful, because the journey process moves you at a level below your everyday awareness. In fact you can't really do this journey wrong. (For additional information on inner journeying, see Sandra Ingerman's book *Shamanic Journeying: A Beginner's Guide*.)

Here are a few guidelines that can help you engage fully in the process, return safely, and trust what is revealed to you.

The music, the voice, the drum

I always use sound to help women on their journey to the Keeper. I'm not talking about background music. I mean sound that is intrinsic to the process, that activates your intuition and creative, quantum thinking. Sound healer and psychologist Tom Kenyon writes eloquently about the transformative effects of the human voice, drums, and flutes. They engage the right side of the brain and increase the theta activity connected with trance states and extraordinary insight. They also signal our left-brain that it's okay to back off for a while. Which is appropriate, because the journey process occurs at a level of our consciousness where linear logic no longer rules. This is a place where paradox is the norm, where animals talk, where gold runs through your veins, where you can crawl into goddesses' wombs, and where the advice offered is probably not what your third-grade teacher gave you. It's an over-the-rainbow place, with its own system of reason. Call it Oz, call it Wonderland, call it Narnia or a wrinkle in time. Shamans call it dreamtime. It's also the place of sexual ecstasy and magic—at the very center of the ISIS Wheel.

Indigenous cultures the world over use drumming as vital to their spiritual journeys and rituals. Rhythmic drumming can promote mystical experiences well beyond your ordinary patterns of organizing information.

This fact is even respected in some scientific circles. Harvard researcher Herbert Benson recognizes the brain-altering quality of rhythmic drumming and uses it as a basis for his best-selling books on relaxation response. Drumming is one of the triggers for what he calls a "breakout" experience to maximize creativity and personal well-being.

The drum I now use for the journey to the Keeper was made by a native Micmac elder near Halifax, Nova Scotia. They say a drum finds you—and this one did, on a spiritual journey I took to Cape Breton Island to celebrate my sixty-fifth birthday. It's also said that the voice of the drum is the heartbeat of Mother Earth—and this is how I experience it. To me, its energy comes straight from Pachamama, the powerful Inca guardian of the earth who absorbs our doubts and fears and returns them to us as wisdom.

All this is to say that journeying to the sound of the drum can be a powerful way to open your ISIS awareness and help you transform how you view your sexual being. You can find CDs of shamanic drumming through the Foundation for Shamanic Studies: www.shamanism.org. You may prefer other kinds of sound. I also use Tibetan bells and flute music, especially the Native American flute, a simple wood instrument that has an otherworldly quality. What's important is to find the kind of sound you like and one that brings you into contact with your deepest self.

Setting the scene for your journey

There are a variety of ways to set the scene for your journey to the Keeper of the Flame. You can light candles, lie around on pillows, drape yourself with silky scarves. You can move and dance. Make your preparations as sensual as you wish. The chapter on ceremony may give you additional ideas for setting the scene. The main thing is to be comfortable, and to imagine these journeys as a form of making love—making love with the universe. Imagine this as a time when you can shed your skin and rebirth yourself to a new look, a new history, a new life.

Clearing your energy

Before any spiritual ritual, it's necessary to clear yourself of your dense, stuck energy (we all have some, unless we're angels), so that you're open to communicating with subtler energy, more light. For ideas on clearing energy, look at the chapter on ceremony. I routinely incorporate a short clearing journey as a kind of a warm-up to the longer journey to your Keeper. It's a meditation that's accompanied by music or drums.

Always, with women's sexuality issues, I find it's crucial to start from a place of safety. That way if you find yourself plunging back into a scary past, or you're not so sure you like the story that's unfolding for you, you can retrace your steps and start again—or just open your eyes and stop.

- Close your eyes and follow your breath inside yourself. Go to a place in your imagination that feels safe. Perhaps this is a place you know well, or perhaps it's new for you. Is it indoors, or outdoors? In the city or in nature? How big is it? How do you feel as you walk around in it? Be aware of the sights, sounds, smells, and textures of this place. Be aware of your breathing.
- Now become aware of your energy. What burdens are you carrying around? What do you need to do to clear your energy for the spiritual journey you're about to undertake? Perhaps you need to bathe in a waterfall. Or burn off some negativity with fire. Or simply brush your skin with your hands. Whatever you need to do, let yourself do it in your imagination and see what happens.
- Allow five minutes or so of music or drumbeats to experience your energy clearing.
- When you're ready, come back into the here and now. Wiggle your fingers and toes and open your eyes. Breathe.
- Take a few minutes to write your experiences, or share them with a partner.

It amazes me how many different ways women find to clear themselves in their imaginations. Everything from sage smoke to bubblebaths and upscale spa treatments. One ISIS woman saw herself being rained on by rose petals. Another had a vision of a red-tailed hawk that soared from the sky and cleared her energy by flapping its wings all over her body.

Contacting your Keeper of the Flame

Now you're ready for the meditative journey to meet your inner guide.

- *Close your eyes, follow your breath inside yourself, to a safe place.* From your place of safety, begin to walk deeper inside to a place that is the source of your sexual energy. Maybe you've been here before, or maybe this is the very first time for you. Maybe the place surprises you. Be aware of what it's like—look, listen, smell, feel—and be aware of your breathing.
- *As you move around in this place, notice that a being appears before you.* The being may be familiar to you, or this may be your very first meeting. Whatever your experience, you instantly recognize this being as the Keeper of the Flame of your sexual energy. Greet each other—and notice what this feels like.
- *Ask this being to accompany you on your journey to sexual wholeness during which you will receive a gift that holds special significance for your ISIS consciousness.* Your gift may appear instantaneously, as it did for the journalist whose story is above. Or it may take a while. In the journey state, clock time is irrelevant.
- *Allow five minutes or longer of music or drumbeats to follow your inner journey.* Let your journey take its natural course. When you receive your gift, recognize how it is important for your ISIS consciousness. Women have received messages of instruction, a sense of belonging, a new identity, and visions of new partners. One woman received an envelope in her father's handwriting and took it as a sign that it was time for her to move beyond her abusive family messages and create loving respect for her sexual self.)
- *When you're ready, find a way to thank your Keeper of the Flame.* And find a way to say good-bye, knowing that you can return whenever you want.
- *Place your gift in a special pocket next to your heart and begin to make your way back through your body and into the here and now.* Wiggle your fingers and toes and open your eyes so that you know you're awake and

fully aware of your surroundings. (Some journeys are so compelling that it's difficult to come back.) Be aware of your breathing.

- Take a few minutes to write down your experiences, or share them with a partner.

End with appreciation and gratitude

Always end your journey with appreciation and gratitude. Praise yourself. Praise your partner, and anyone else who may have been involved in this journey. Praise the spirits of insight, complexity, creativity, and courage. If "nothing" seemed to happen, praise the spirits of silence, of blank pages, of enveloping mists and clouds of poignant emptiness. Most of all, sing praises for allowing yourself to embark on this special journey to the heart and soul of sex.

EPILOGUE

Making Peace with Our Bodies

IN RESPONSE TO THE terrorist attacks on the glittering blue and gold morning of September 11, 2001, I turned off the TV images of destruction and drove to the ocean to seek comfort and grounding. Within the hour I was at Singing Beach in Manchester, Massachusetts, which holds deeply nurturing little-girl memories for me. I'd learned to swim there. I'd eaten Fluffernutters and built sand castles there, always knowing that by morning the surf would have swallowed every trace of what I'd built and returned it to the wide sweep of shoreline. As I stumbled onto the beach, I heard a cry of agony. I realized it was my own: *"What am I doing researching sexuality and spirituality when all these really important events are happening in the world—?"*

As so often happens when the time is ripe, the answer came back fully formed even before I'd completed the question. *"Your job is to teach about nonviolent relationships,"* the ocean boomed. *"Now get back there and get on with it!"*

I was able to put this commandment into action that very weekend when I was conducting a workshop at Rowe Conference Center in the Berkshires. The 9/11 energy impelled our circle of women to ask the big questions about sexual desire and partnership: What *are* love and sex? What do they mean in our lives? How do our yearnings for belonging and pleasure connect to the sweep of world events?

Together we explored the notion that our intimate relationships form a template for all the relationships that affect our lives. That is, how each of us relates with our bodies, ourselves, and our partners lays down the basic pattern for how we relate with our families, our coworkers, our communities, and beyond, including politics, the environment, and even the realm of spirit—God, Goddess, Higher Power, Universal Energy. Simply stated, all of these relationships begin at home, in our hearts, minds, and bodies. Self-acceptance and love lead to growthful, soulful connections. Fear and self-hatred lead to control, alienation, and violence. Riane Eisler lays out these ideas with grace and brilliance in her book *The Power of Partnership*.

Once we accept that our personal ecosystems are part of a very much larger picture, it's possible to envision how each one of us affects the collective reality. If we believe that pleasure is an integral part of the colorful mandala of creation, nurturing our bodies can become an act of worship. And it can become an act of resilience and optimism to ally our physical bodies with the energies beyond—the unseen world inhabited by powerful spirits, who really do guide our steps when we let go and let them.

The present turmoil in the world presents a prime opportunity to exercise our ordinary and extraordinary abilities for such connection. We can begin by resisting images of war and destruction and make peace with our own bodies. The winter before we bombed Baghdad, some hardy women in a handful of communities around the globe chose to take this idea literally. They stripped off their clothes and spelled out P-E-A-C-E with their naked bodies. But we can participate at other levels, too, fully clothed, as long as we are also fully aware.

To prepare the template of inner peace, it may be necessary to unlearn old fears, old pain, old images, old ways of holding on to what's no longer useful—workaholism, victim roles, just-say-no messages. We can allow ourselves to feel deeply connected to the earth and to all the beings, seen and unseen, who inhabit it. Once we've experienced that knowing in our cells, we can never be at a total loss, even when the world around us seems to be spinning out of control.

Walking this path of connection means surrendering the defenses we've constructed around our bodies, minds, and emotions so that the flow of spirit can enter in. How do we surrender these defenses? Breathe—this is inspiration at its most literal. And when we breathe together it becomes *con*spiracy. Trust—hold the energy of yes instead of no. Expand the heart in love. Ask for help with an open hand. Sing the sudden music of praise. Or (perhaps most radically) stop doing. Simply hold space and allow the cycles of nature to work their magic, as they did on my sand castles so long ago. In

the words of a wise Buddhist friend, "Don't just do something. Sit there."
This, too, can fulfill the injunction about nonviolent relationships so clearly
communicated to me on 9/11 and still so poignant in the years since.

It's customary to begin a spiritual journey with an offering. But in this
book I would like to end with an offering—a kind of love poem. This is a
prayer for new endings and new beginnings, an invocation to the spirits in
time of national neurosis and international fear. I've addressed it to "a
woman," but it's intended for all who feel a connection with it.

FOR A WOMAN WHO FEARS SHE
IS TOO DAMAGED TO LOVE AGAIN

Holy spirits of fire befriend and warm this woman.
Earth and water wrap her in bounty.
Spirits of air guide her to walk the paths of her heart.

Sun smile on her. Stones accept her. Stars remind her.
Ocean storms burnish her terrors to translucent pearls.
Creatures of hills and hollows, beings beneath the ground
watch over her, comfort and nourish her.
Snakes and rivers, ancient dragons dance sinuously with her.
Swirling spirit of volcano invest her with power.
Eagle and sparrow give her wings and sight.

Snails of Buddha, saints of God, Great Spirit
Yahweh, Magus, Shiva, Isis, Astarte of the flowing hair,
Goddess of Grain, Angel of Sweetness, Higher Power,
protect this fearful one, this angry, armored one,
this giver, healer, striver, survivor, lover.
Cherish her—waif and victim, elf and Amazon.
See this holy woman now. Touch her.
Brush her with the breath of love.

Ganesh, sacred elephant who cries human tears
and oversees new ventures, help her begin again.

ACKNOWLEDGMENTS

IT'S TAKEN A GOOD-SIZED village to bring this book into being. Now it's my delight to go door-to-door with bouquets of thanks. First and most profound gratitude goes to the 3,810 survey respondents who are at the heart and soul of this book. I know size isn't everything, but your response was huge as well as eloquent, and demonstrates that the ISIS connection is an idea whose time has come.

Next, I thank my agent, Ellen Levine, for connecting me with Shambhala, whose books are wise and beautiful. Equally deep appreciation to my editor, Eden Steinberg, who is the spirit of insight and collaboration.

I think of Riane Eisler as the intellectual mother of this book, for she has given generously of her time to help it grow from the very first seedling of an idea in 1995. Christiane Northrup and Judy Norsigian each offered wonderful opportunities for me to reach out to their extensive networks of women. Many other colleagues also took time from their own endeavors to support this project, and it seemed that whenever something was needed, the right person appeared.

For guiding me through the mysteries of survey design and the statistical mazes of sexual science I'm indebted to Judy Bradford, Carol Ellison, Robert Hawkins, David Kahn, Peggy Kleinplatz, Patricia Koch, Barry Komisaruk, Jennifer Moye, Jean Powell, Louise Rice, Deborah Tolman, Douglas Wallace, Beverly Whipple, and Elaine Young.

For enthusiasm and goodwill, piloting and distributing the ISIS survey, entering data, compiling information, and helping me understand (and find ways to talk about) the historical, social, religious, medical, political, environmental, and gender-bending contexts of both sex and spirit, I thank Deborah Anapol, Shirley Anderson, Roberta Antoniotti, Prue Berry, Kate Bornstein, Robert Bridges, Patti Britton, Leslie Brunetta, Shawna Carroll,

Debra Cash, Carol Caton, Rebecca Chalker, Maureen Chase, Susan Chiatt, Jane Claypool, Ani Colt, Annie Cotten, Maril Crabtree, Joy Davidson, Katja Esser, David Farkas, Sallie Foley, Robert Francoeur, Robert Friar, Ellen Friedman, Elinor Gadon, Emily Godfrey, Judy Hancock, Bernardine Hayes, Fran Henry, Karen Hicks, Peggy Huddleston, Mary Hunt, Loraine Hutchins, Constance Jones, Ari Kane, Adele Kennedy (rest in peace, dear Adele), Peggy Kleinplatz, Pam Kramer, Mary Krueger, Jackie Lapidus, Eve LaPlante, Sally Lehr, Gail Leondar-Wright, David Loye, Karen MacArthur, Wendy Maltz, Ron Mazur, Ruth McConnell, Karen McDaniel, Mary Mumford, Alexandra Myles, Judy Peres, Carole Rayburn, Jane Redmont, Cintra Reeve, Suzann Robins, Janis Roihl, Deborah Rose, Deloris Roys, Howard Ruppell, Nannette Sawyer, Sandra Scantling, Ilene Serlin, Julian Slowinski, Elena Stone, Kenneth Ray Stubbs, Mitchell Tepper, Leonore Tiefer, Joan Timmerman, Jean Trounstine, Judy Tsukroff, Dell Williams, Jean Winslow, and Stephanie Young.

Joan Duncan Oliver, then editor-in-chief of *New Age* magazine, recognized the unique nature of the ISIS survey and arranged to have the questionnaire published for readers to fill out. Six months later, Laura Ziv arranged for publication of the ISIS survey in *New Woman* magazine, where she was an editor. Your leaps of faith gave thousands of readers permission to tell their stories, which have immeasurably enriched this book.

The Radcliffe Institute honored me with a year as a visiting scholar to analyze the survey results (1999–2000). My special appreciation to Barbara Haber for sponsoring me at the Schlesinger Library, where I had the opportunity to evaluate the ISIS findings in one of the great bastions of women's history. Thanks to Rodney Glasgow and Katherine Quible, my research assistants while I was there, to Akinyi Opeyo, who helped me sort out ISIS statistics, and to Sarah Gibb, who interned with me the following year to analyze the ISIS data on spirituality and religion.

The Wellesley Centers for Research on Women honored me with a year as a visiting scholar to report on the survey results (2001–2002). Special thanks to Deborah Tolman and Sumru Erkut for sponsoring me, and to Michelle Porche, Cassandra Kisiel, and Linda Gardiner for careful peer review of the initial ISIS report. For wisdom and encouragement I'm also grateful to Ruth Harriet Jacobs, Hilda Gaspar-Periera, and my ongoing scholarly lunch mates, Ruth Hannon and Jane Wegscheider Hyman.

In 2002, Susan Sered invited me to join her remarkable Women Healing Women program at the Harvard Divinity School's Center for the Study of World Religions. I am especially grateful to her for helping me obtain a grant to explore sexual issues for menopausal women—a study that will inform the third book in this Shambhala series. Also thanks to the Foundation for the Scientific Study of Sexuality for funding a study on the multidimensionality of meaningful sexual experience, a theme that is basic to this book.

A group of spiritually focused sexuality educators, therapists, and physicians met monthly at my house in 2002 and 2003 to discuss the earliest drafts of what was to morph into this book. Hilary Graham, Anne Hallward, Irene Monroe, Jennifer Moye, Camilla Opeyemi Parham, Meg Striepe, and Rosemary Rossi shored up my confidence in the ISIS material when I most needed it, and helped shape the tone and direction this book has taken—thank you.

Through seemingly endless versions of the book proposal I was blessed with graceful insights from five extraordinary authors. Profound thanks to Joan Duncan Oliver, Sarah Wernick, Judith Nies, Lynda Morgenroth, and Amy Hoffman—kindred spirits all.

Rowe Conference Center has offered me an open-hearted forum over the years in which to present ISIS workshops—which I continue to colead with Prue Berry. For other forums in which to present the ISIS findings and receive valuable feedback from a wide range of professionals and nonprofessionals, I thank the American Association of Sex Educators, Counselors and Therapists; the American Psychological Association; the American Public Health Association; the Association for Women in Psychology; Esalen Institute; the Fenway Institute; the Gerontological Society of America; Harvard Divinity School's Center for the Study of World Religions; Interface Foundation; the International Association for the Study of Dreams; the International Society for the Study of Women's Sexual Health; the Institute for Twenty-first Century Relationships; Lesley University's Spirituality Institute; the National Women's Health Network; the New View Campaign; Planned Parenthood Federation of America;

the Radcliffe Institute; Simmons College; the Society for the Scientific Study of Sexuality; the Theological Opportunities Program; the Wellesley Centers for Research on Women; and the Women's Well.

My enduring gratitude to the healers, teachers, and ceremonialists who nurtured my body, mind, heart, and spirit during these ten years, especially Reva Seybolt, Oscar Miro-Quesada, Emilie Conrad, Ilene Myers, Lydia Knudson, Lynn Abbott, Maribeth Kaptchuk, Nina Murphy, Jeanne Hubbuch, and Donna Fayad. Thanks also to Addie Escarcida, intrepid "computer whisperer," who saved the ISIS data from a near-death experience in 2001 and has kept my laptop up and running ever since.

To dear ones who've fed me, inspired me, and otherwise nourished me with friendship, comfort, play, music, ceremony, travel, and memories that fill my heart—Prue Berry, Mary Bewig, Sandy Bierig, Peggy Clark, Ani Colt, Maril Crabtree, Ruth Fishel, Karen Hicks, Barbara Lambert, Alexandra Myles, Judith Nies, Deborah Rose, Pepita Seth, Anne Stone, and Anne Zevin. To Kaye Andres, who left her body in April 2005—your spirit infuses this book.

To my daughter, Cathy Saunders, and son, Philip Saunders—I am so deeply moved by the amazing and generous people you've become despite my parenting blunders, and to my daughter-in-law, Wendy Saunders, whose heart is as open as the ocean. To my grandchildren, Christopher and Christina—you are the future and you are filled with light.

The biggest, most lavish bouquet of all belongs to Jo Chaffee, for twenty-five years my loving partner and meticulous first editor. This book would never be without you.

INTEGRATING SEXUALITY
AND SPIRITUALITY

A Survey

THIS IS THE ISIS survey with the questions answered by all 3,810 respondents. Percentages are in round numbers and may not add up exactly to 100 percent. Some survey questions invited respondents to check more than one alternative, and may add to more than 100 percent. For an analysis of ISIS answers by respondents' gender, sexual preference, spiritual orientation, religion, and so on, please contact me through my website: www.GinaOgden.com.

Although I am not collecting new ISIS data at this time, you may want to complete the survey to find out how you answer the questions. Note what questions you have problems answering, and what questions you might add to the survey. Taking the survey with your partner can open new areas of sexual communication. The survey questions can also be instructive for students, clients, and colleagues. You can download a blank survey from my website.

1. **Age** 18–86 **Gender** Female 82% Male 18% Crossgender <1%
   Occupation businesspeople 35% students 18% professionals 16%
   manual laborers 10% homemakers 5%

2. **Area you live in** Every state in the U.S.

3. **Highest education completed** 1 Grade School 3% 2 High School 32%
   3 College 42% 4 Master's 19% 5 Doctorate 3% 6 Post Doctorate 1%

4. **Ethnic identification** 1 Caucasian (White) 86% 2 African-American (Black) 4%
   3 Hispanic 3% 4 Native American 1% 5 Asian <1% 6 Multiethnic 5%

5. **Yearly household income** Average $55,770

6. **Religion you grew up with** 1 Roman Catholic 39% 2 Protestant 34%
   3 Fundamentalist Christian 7% 4 Jewish 5% 5 Buddhist <1% 6 Mormon 1%
   7 Atheist 1% 8 Agnostic 4% 9 None 3% 10 Other 5%

7. **Religious affiliation now** 1 Roman Catholic 19% 2 Protestant 20%
   3 Fundamentalist Christian 5% 4 Jewish 3% 5 Buddhist 3% 6 Mormon 1%
   7 Atheist 2% 8 Agnostic 3% 9 None 24% 10 Other 21%

8. **Political philosophy** 1 Liberal 60% 2 Conservative 19% 3 Other 21%

9. **Attitude toward abortion** 1 Pro-choice 80% 2 Anti-Abortion 14% 3 Other 6%

10. **Sexual preference** 1 Heterosexual 80% 2 Bisexual 7% 3 Lesbian/Gay 5%

11. **Relationship status** 1 No current partner 17% 2 Married 18% 3 In a
    committed relationship 18% 4 Separated 2% 5 Divorced 4% 6 Widowed 1%

12. **Number of years (or fraction of years) with current partner** Average 5½ years

13. **Disabilities/chronic illnesses** 1 Cancer 1% 2 Heart Disease 1%
    3 HIV/AIDS <1% 4 Diabetes 2% 5 Arthritis 3% 6 Depression 19%
    7 None 73% 8 Other 1%

14. **Experience of sexual abuse** 1 As a child 25% 2 As an adult 13% 3 Never 75%

15. **Addictive use of alcohol and/or drugs** 1 In the past 18% 2 In the present 4%
    3 Never 78%

16. **Here are some comments people have made about sex and spirituality.** (check all that reflect your experience)

   1 39% "Sex usually means intercourse."

   2 78% "For me, sex is much more than intercourse; it involves all of me—body, mind, heart, and soul."

   3 10% "I associate spirituality mainly with going to church."

   4 55% "When I open myself to warmth, desire, depth, expansion, and trust, there is no separation between sex and spirit."

   5 3% "Sex is for conceiving babies and has little to do with spirituality."

   6 45% "It's through my senses that I often experience God."

   7 8% "All my life I've been told that people who love sex *too much* will go to hell."

   8 51% "Mainly, sex means connection with my partner."

   9 85% "Sex is physical, but it also involves love, romance, even mystical union."

   10 47% "For people who have been sexually disappointed or hurt, consciously giving and receiving sexual pleasure can be healing."

17. **Sexual romance and religious worship have many kinds of symbols and rituals in common.** (check *all* that you associate with *both* your sexuality *and* your spirituality)

1 82% Candles		7 30% Special foods
2 47% Incense		8 70% Words of comfort
3 64% Flowers		9 83% Words of love
4 47% Wine		10 51% Laying on of hands
5 82% Music		11 3% None of the above
6 47% Dancing		12 13% Other

18. **When I use the word "spirituality" in the context of my sexuality, I mean:** (check one)

   1 70% Spirituality but not religion

   2 4% Religion but not spirituality

   3 21% Spirituality and religion combined

   4 5% Other

19. **To me, it seems sacrilegious to talk about sex and spirituality together.**
   1 Yes 9%   2 No 91%

. . . survey continued next page

20. What do sexuality and spirituality involve in your life?

SEXUALITY INVOLVES

97% Excitement	....	Boredom 2%
94% Honesty	....	Deception 3%
78% Caring for others	....	Caring for self 10%
46% Numbed senses	....	Heightened senses 47%
95% Intense body pleasure	....	Minimal body pleasure 2%
91% Intense inner vitality	....	Minimal inner vitality 5%
46% Constraint	....	Liberation 45%
92% Integration	....	Fragmentation 3%
90% Oneness with self	....	Distance from self 2%
94% Oneness with partner	....	Distance from partner 3%
83% Oneness with a power greater than self	....	Distance from a power 7% greater than self
84% Worship	....	Blasphemy 4%
92% Other		

SPIRITUALITY INVOLVES

91% Excitement	....	Boredom 3%
97% Honesty	....	Deception <1%
78% Caring for others	....	Caring for self 13%
45% Numbed senses	....	Heightened senses 47%
66% Intense body pleasure	....	Minimal body pleasure 19%
90% Intense inner vitality	....	Minimal inner vitality 5%
46% Constraint	....	Liberation 45%
93% Integration	....	Fragmentation 3%
93% Oneness with self	....	Distance from self 3%
85% Oneness with partner	....	Distance from partner 6%
96% Oneness with a power greater than self	....	Distance from a power 1% greater than self
95% Worship	....	Blasphemy 1%
94% Other		

21. Which *one* of the above statements would you say is *most* true?
    1 of your current sexual experience? oneness with partner (15%)
    2 of your current spiritual experience? oneness with greater power (18%)

22. **Sex needs to have a spiritual element to be really satisfying.** (check one)
    1 Always true for me 26%
    2 Sometimes true for me 43%
    3 Neither true nor untrue for me 21%
    4 Seldom true for me 4%
    5 Never true for me 4%

23. **With which of the following has sex been a spiritual experience for you?** (check *all* that apply)
    1 Husband 38% (of women)
    2 Wife 40% (of men)
    3 Committed partner 58%
    4 Casual encounter 19%
    5 Affair while committed to someone else 15%
    6 Self 21%

24. **Sex has been *most* spiritual with which partner in question 23?**
    committed partner (43%)

25. **Sex has been *least* spiritual with which partner in question 23?**
    casual partner (26%)

26. **Which of the following have contributed to sex being a spiritual experience for you?** (check *all* that apply)
    1 Being in love 81%
    2 Conceiving a baby 41%
    3 Being pregnant 33%
    4 Having no fear of getting pregnant 38%
    5 Feeling committed to my partner 52%
    6 Feeling free of responsibility to my partner 14%

. . . survey continued next page

7   Feeling safe 59%

8   Experiencing a personal crisis 33%

9   Feeling in control 44%

10 Feeling controlled 24%

11 Being in the mood 38%

12 Aggressive thrusting 22%

13 Danger 30%

14 Drinking or drugs 32%

15 None of the above 8%

16 Other 13%

27. **Which** *one* **of the above circumstances has contributed** *most* **to spiritual sex?**
being in love (44%)

28. **Which** *one* **of the above circumstances has contributed** *least* **to spiritual sex?**
drinking or drugs (15%) feeling controlled (12%) danger (12%)

29. **Which of the following have you done to help bring a spiritual dimension to your sexual experiences?** (check *all* that apply)

1 Made eye contact with
   my partner 77%

2 Shared deep feelings with
   my partner 79%

3 Lit candles or incense 64%

4 Bathed together 57%

5 Enjoyed special foods 30%

6 Meditated before
   getting physical 16%

7 Made love in a special place 46%

8 Touched reverently 66%

9 Kissed soulfully 79%

10 Played music 24%

11 Danced 38%

12 Fantasized or daydreamed 43%

13 Laughed together 71%

14 Let go of control 60%

15 Did nothing special 15%

16 Other 81%

30. **Which** *one* **of the above choices has been** *most* **helpful in bringing a spiritual dimension to your sexuality?** sharing deep feelings (33%)

31. **Which** *one* **of the above choices has been** *least* **helpful in bringing a spiritual dimension to your sexuality?** doing nothing special (15%) special foods (14%)

32. **How have your spiritual beliefs led you to express your sexuality more fully?** (check *all* that apply)

    1   By affirming that love is good in all its forms and expressions 72%

    2   By teaching that making love is holy 29%

    3   By opening me to risk deeper intimacy 57%

    4   By giving me faith when I've felt like running away from pleasure 27%

    5   By sanctioning my feelings of longing and passion 37%

    6   By making the physical part of relationship into a sacrament 27%

    7   Other 9%

33. **How have your spiritual beliefs prevented you from expressing your sexuality as fully as you might?** (check *all* that apply)

    1   By giving me the message "good girls don't" 32%

    2   By making sexual desire a source of guilt 32%

    3   By making the body a source of shame 23%

    4   By teaching that sex is not for pleasure, but for procreation (conceiving babies) 13%

    5   By teaching that pleasure is more important for a man than for a woman 18%

    6   By keeping me from exploring sexual taboos 31%

    7   Other 15%

34. **Has anything else in your life prevented you from experiencing a sex-spirit connection?** (check *all* that apply)

1 Childhood abuse 22%	11 My partner only thinking about physical kicks 20%
2 Abuse as an adult 15%	12 Not loving my partner 28%
3 Drinking and/or drug use 15%	13 My partner not loving me 26%
4 Depression and/or anxiety 39%	14 Sex isn't that interesting to me 8%
5 Physical disabilities 6%	15 Spirituality isn't that interesting to me 4%
6 Worry about how I look 47%	16 I've never thought of spirituality as a part of sex before now 15%
7 Getting older 13%	17 Other 14%
8 Not having a partner 29%	
9 Pregnancy 6%	
10 Parenthood 9%	

. . . survey continued next page

35. Which *one* of the above choices has *most* prevented you from experiencing a sex-spirit connection? worry about how I look (11%) not loving partner (10%) childhood abuse (9%)

36. Have you ever experienced sexual ecstasy? 1 Yes 84%   2 No 13%

37. Have you ever experienced spiritual ecstasy? 1 Yes 70%   2 No 27%

38.–39. Some people feel that experiences they associate with sexual satisfaction are similar to experiences they associate with spiritual satisfaction. What do you associate with your sexual satisfaction and/or spiritual satisfaction? (check *all* that apply)

	38. ASSOCIATE WITH SEXUAL SATISFACTION		39. ASSOCIATE WITH SPIRITUAL SATISFACTION	
Release of body tension	1	91%	1	56%
Release of emotional tension	2	80%	2	79%
Heightened senses	3	80%	3	68%
Clarity of understanding	4	36%	4	82%
Surge of energy	5	72%	5	59%
Peace and serenity	6	67%	6	89%
Feeling loved and accepted	7	85%	7	77%
Feeling loving and accepting	8	79%	8	77%
Oneness with self	9	55%	9	78%
Oneness with partner	10	84%	10	49%
Oneness with nature	11	38%	11	75%
Oneness with a power greater than self	12	37%	12	81%
Other (please specify)	13	8%	13	6%

40. Which one of the above experiences is *most* essential to your *sexual* satisfaction? feeling loved and accepted (32%)

41. Which one of the above experiences is *most* essential to your *spiritual* satisfaction? oneness with a power greater than self (30%)

42. In a moment of *sexual* ecstasy have you ever had a sense of experiencing God/Universal Energy? 1 Yes 47%   2 No 49%

43. In a moment of *spiritual* ecstasy have you ever felt a surge of sexual energy?
    1 Yes 45%   2 No 47%

44. Please indicate how important the following concepts are for your present life situation.

	IMPORTANT	NOT IMPORTANT
1 Sexuality	84%	14%
2 Spirituality	91%	10%
3 Religion	34%	59%

(optional)

Below or on a separate piece of paper please tell us more about your sexuality and spirituality. How did you discover that sex can be spiritual? What are your most memorable experiences—by yourself and/or with a partner?

1,465 respondents (38% of the total ISIS sample) wrote letters describing their experiences

EXTRAGENITAL MATRIX: SEXUAL ENJOYMENT BEYOND THE USUAL "HOMING SITES"

Rate from 0 to 10 (0 not at all, 10 ecstatic) how much you enjoy various kinds of touch on different parts of your body

	KINDS OF TOUCH Touching by hand			
WHERE ON MY BODY	SOFT STROKING	DEEP STROKING	RUBBING	PATTING
Head and Face				
Hair/Scalp				
Cheeks				
Lips				
Ears				
Neck and Torso				
Neck				
Shoulders				
Stomach				
Back				
Buttocks				
Arms and Hands				
Arms				
Elbows				
Wrists				
Palms				
Fingers				
Legs and Feet				
Legs				
Ankles				
Feet				
Toes				
Full Body				
Other				

EXTRAGENITAL MATRIX

	KISSING	LICKING	SUCKING	NIPPING	
KINDS OF TOUCH **Touching by mouth**					
					WHERE ON MY BODY
					Head and Face
					Hair/Scalp
					Cheeks
					Lips
					Ears
					Neck and Torso
					Neck
					Shoulders
					Stomach
					Back
					Buttocks
					Arms and Hands
					Arms
					Elbows
					Wrists
					Palms
					Fingers
					Legs and Feet
					Legs
					Ankles
					Feet
					Toes
					Full Body
					Other

RESOURCES FOR BRINGING
MORE HEART AND SOUL INTO
YOUR SEXUAL EXPERIENCES

AFTER READING THIS book you may feel you want more—more conversation, more education, perhaps even professional training in how you can broaden your definitions of sex and integrate sexuality and spirituality in your life.

For more information about the ISIS survey, visit my website: www.GinaOgden.com. You'll find a survey questionnaire you can download, lots of ISIS facts and numbers that wouldn't fit in this book, an ISIS discussion guide, a bibliography, articles by me and by other experts on women's sexual relationships, and links to informative websites. You'll also find a calendar of my presentations and workshops, and you can communicate directly with me through my website, so I invite you to check it out!

Listed below are other websites that can help you expand your thinking and connect you with other people exploring similar paths.

ISIS CONNECTION GROUPS

Several healers around the country are offering ISIS Connection groups to discuss the concepts in this book and how to put them into practice. For information on these groups, or how to start your own group, see my website, www.GinaOgden.com

Information on Women's Health and Sexual Health

Planned Parenthood Federation of America (www.ppfa.org)
Planned Parenthood operates nearly 850 health centers in forty-nine states and the District of Columbia. They provide culturally sensitive pro-choice sexuality information and counseling to millions of women, men, and teenagers each year regardless of race, age, disability, sexual orientation, or income. They also offer educational programs for health professionals.

The Sexuality Information and Education Council of the U.S. (www.siecus.org)
This organization, whose acronym is SIECUS, offers a comprehensive list of sexuality education books and pamphlets, along with bibliographies arranged by various topics. SIECUS has developed the National School Health Clearinghouse to give professionals easy access to essential information for young people. Much of the SIECUS material can be downloaded free.

Our Bodies, Ourselves (www.ourbodiesourselves.org)
This is the public interest advocacy group that created the best-selling *Our Bodies, Ourselves* and inspired the women's health movement in the 1970s. The website serves as a multicultural health information center for women, with excerpts from the book and links to additional information. Spanish-language translations are available for much of the information.

The National Women's Health Network (www.womenshealthnetwork.org)
This is a membership-based organization whose aim is to give women a greater voice within the health care system. The website offers information on issues that shape the major health decisions of women of all sexual orientations, races, and socioeconomic circumstances.

Go Ask Alice (www.goaskalice.columbia.edu)
This is the Internet service of Columbia University's Health Services program. It's a resource for everyone who wants to ask a question or read the answers. The website provides reliable information and a range of perspectives about relationships; sexuality; sexual health; emotional health; fitness; nutrition; alcohol, nicotine, and other drugs; and general health.

The National Gay and Lesbian Task Force (www.thetaskforce.org)
This is a major website that connects lesbian, gay, bisexual, and transgender communities in the United States. It links to many local resources that cover everything from coming out to how to have safe—and spiritual—sexual relationships.

Bisexual Resource Center (www.biresource.org)
This is the most comprehensive resource for information on bisexual lifestyles, bi-related events, books, videos, and recordings.

The New View of Women's Sexuality (www.fsd-alert.org)
This innovative educational resource looks beyond pharmaceutical interventions for "female sexual dysfunction" (FSD) to view the emotional and social complexities involved in women's sexual problems—and pleasures.

The Women's Sexual Health Foundation (www.twshf.org)
This organization focuses on the medical treatment of sexual problems, but also supports a multidisciplinary approach to sexual health. The website includes surveys and suggested readings.

Stop It Now (www.stopitnow.org)
This is an innovative program whose aim is to prevent child sexual abuse through public education rather than only punishing the offenders. Its website offers information to people concerned about inappropriate sexualized behavior in adults, adolescents, or children, and to people concerned about their own sexual thoughts or behaviors.

WEBSITES BY SEXUALITY EXPERTS

Many sexuality experts have developed their own educational websites. I'm able to include only a few here, but if you're interested in other experts cited in this book, chances are a Google search will turn up their sites. The websites below are designed to help people of all ages and sexual orientations understand and enjoy meaningful sexual experience that is based on caring, respect, health, and intimacy.

The Sexual Health Network (www.sexualhealth.com)

Dr. Mitchell Tepper has created this comprehensive website, which is devoted to sexuality issues of all kinds, and is the best resource I know for people with disabilities. It, too, includes an extensive bibliography.

College Sex Talk (www.collegesextalk.com)

Professor Sandra Caron is the syndicated columnist for this interactive site where young people can ask questions and receive thoughtful answers on subjects that range from safe sex to sexual orientation.

The Religious Institute (www.religiousinstitute.org)

Reverend Debra Haffner has created this site as an expression of religion, sexual morality, justice, and healing—the need for a sexual ethic that's based on relationship rather than on specific sex acts.

Wendy Maltz (www.healthysex.com)

Therapist and author Wendy Maltz is the creator of this site, which offers information, books, and videos on aspects of sexuality that range from the pleasures of fantasy to healing from abuse and violence.

Betty Dodson (www.bettydodson.com)

Sex educator Betty Dodson has been teaching the health and joys of masturbation since the early 1970s. Her website is irreverent, educational—and explicit, offering an on-line index to all aspects of self-pleasure, including her own groundbreaking books and videos.

Christiane Northrup (www.drnorthrup.com)
Dr. Christiane Northrup is a pioneer in mind-body health and well-being for women. This website gives you access to her philosophy and to her information-packed monthly e-newsletter.

EDUCATIONAL OPPORTUNITIES

There are numerous ways you can learn more about the heart and soul of sex. Where you might start depends on your income, your level of interest, and how far you want to travel—both geographically and on your life's path.

Workshops

You can take workshops for a day, a weekend, or more that will connect you with gifted teachers and with participants who are moved to follow this path. There are wonderful, vibrant conference centers and holistic learning centers around the country. Each has its own character, so decide if you want an urban experience or a trip to the sea or mountains. Centers I'm most familiar with include:

- Esalen Institute in Big Sur, California, www.esalen.org
- Kripalu Center in Lenox, Massachusetts, www.kripalu.org
- New York Open Center in New York City, www.opencenter.org
- Omega Institute in Rhinebeck, New York, www.eomega.org
- Rowe Conference Center in Rowe, Massachusetts, www.rowecenter.org
- Women's Well in West Concord, Massachusetts, www.womenswell.org

Two sexuality organizations that have no stay-on-the premises center, but that offer workshops and trainings internationally are:

- The Body Electric School, www.bodyelectric.org
- The Human Awareness Institute, www.hai.org

Professional conferences

Conferences offered by professional organizations focus on scholarly education and training. They also afford a valuable opportunity to network with others engaged in the work. Three of the major sexuality organizations that open their conferences to both professionals and nonprofessionals are:

- The American Association of Sexuality Educators, Counselors, and Therapists (AASECT), www.aasect.org
- The Society for the Scientific Study of Sexuality (SSSS), www.sexscience.org
- The International Society for the Study of Women's Sexual Health (ISSWSH), www.isswsh.org

Colleges and universities

If you feel you want more formal study, you can explore the undergraduate and graduate programs that focus on the interdisciplinary field of human sexuality. You can find a comprehensive list on the SSSS website: www.sexscience.org. The two major degree-granting institutions are:

- The Institute for the Advanced Study of Human Sexuality in San Francisco, California, www.iashs.org
- Widener University Human Sexuality Program, near Philadelphia, Pennsylvania, www.widener.edu

TOYS, DVDS, AND EROTICA—OH MY!

Another way to explore your sexuality is through inventive sex toys and other products that remind you that sex is good, and that connecting yourself body, mind, heart, and soul is even better.

Women's boutiques

There are thousands of online sex stores, but the ISIS recommendations are for boutiques designed especially for women. These are discreet, delightful environments, and if you need assistance, the staffs are generally knowledgeable. You can purchase books and videos along with vibrators and other goodies for enhancing your sexual pleasure. Many of these boutiques offer interesting workshops and other educational opportunities. Their websites and catalogs are an education in themselves.

- Eve's Garden, in New York City, www.evesgarden.com
- Good Vibrations, in San Francisco and Boston, www.goodvibes.com
- Toys in Babeland, in New York and Seattle, www.toysinbabeland.com
- Early to Bed, in Chicago, www.early2bed.com
- Grand Opening, a virtual store at www.grandopening.com

Erotic and educational videos and DVDs
- Femme Productions, www.royalle.com. Candida Royalle owns and runs Femme Productions, which has produced woman-centered erotic films and sex aids for many years.
- The Sinclair Intimacy Institute, www.bettersex.com, provides educational videos that demonstrate explicit sexual techniques. These are often narrated by a sex therapist.
- Secret Garden Publishing, www.secretgardenpublishing.com. Kenneth Ray Stubbs, Ph.D. is a gifted teacher whose thoughtful, beautiful books and DVDs embody the sensual intimacy of women, sex, and spirit.

COUNSELING AND THERAPY (WWW.AASECT.ORG)

The American Association of Sex Educators, Counselors, and Therapists (AASECT) is an interdisciplinary organization that supervises and certifies health professionals all over North America. Its members include physicians, nurses, social workers, psychologists, allied health professionals, clergy members, lawyers, sociologists, marriage and family counselors and therapists, family planning specialists, and researchers. The website provides a database of board-certified sexuality educators, counselors, and therapists, along with certification standards and procedures for sexuality professionals.

SUGGESTED READINGS

BOOKS TO EXPAND YOUR VIEW OF SEXUAL HEALTH AND PLEASURE

Angier, Natalie. *Woman: An Intimate Geography*. Boston: Houghton-Mifflin, 1999.

Boston Women's Health Book Collective. *Our Bodies, Oourselves: A New Edition for a New Era*. New York: Simon and Schuster, 2005.

Chalker, Rebecca. *The Clitoral Truth: The Secret World at Our Fingertips*. New York: Seven Stories Press, 2000.

Cornog, Martha. *The Big Book of Masturbation: From Angst to Zeal*. San Francisco: Down There Press, 2003.

Dodson, Betty. *Sex for One: The Joy of Self-Loving*. Rev. ed. New York: Crown, 1996.

Eisler, Riane. *The Power of Partnership: Seven Relationships That Will Change Your Life*. New York: New World Library, 2002.

Ensler, Eve. *The Vagina Monologues: The V-Day Edition*. New York: Villard, 2000.

Maltz, Wendy and Suzie Boss. *Private Thoughts: Exploring the Power of Women's Sexual Fantasies*. New York: New World Library, 2001.

Ogden, Gina. *Women Who Love Sex: An Inquiry into the Expanding Spirit of Women's Erotic Experience*. Rev. ed. Cambridge, Mass.: Womanspirit Press, 1999.

OUR SEXUAL HISTORY, OUR SEXUAL DIVERSITY

Anapol, Deborah. *Polyamory: The New Love without Limits: Secrets of Sustainable Intimate Relationships*. Rev. ed. San Raphael, Calif.: IntiNet Resource Center, 1997.

Ehrenreich, Barbara. *Witches, Midwives and Nurses: A History of Women Healers.* New York: Feminist Press, 1972.

Espin, Oliva M. *Latina Realities: Essays on Healing, Migration, and Sexuality.* Boulder, Colo., 1997: Westview Press.

Giddings, Paula. *When and Where I Enter: The Impact of Black Women on Race and Sex in America.* New York: William Morrow, 1984.

Hall, Marny. *The Lesbian Love Companion.* San Francisco: Harper San Francisco, 1998.

Hutchins, Loraine, and Lani Kaahumanu, eds. *Bi Any Other Name: Bisexual People Speak Out.* Los Angeles: Alyson Publications, 1991.

Kilbourne, Jean. *Can't Buy My Love: How Advertising Changes the Way We Think and Feel.* New York: Free Press, 2000.

Somé, Sobonfu E. *The Spirit of Intimacy: Ancient Teachings in the Ways of Relationships.* Berkeley, Calif.: Berkeley Hills Books, 1997.

Wyatt, Gail Elizabeth. *Stolen Women: Reclaiming Our Sexuality, Taking Back Our Lives.* New York: John Wiley & Sons, 1997.

PRACTICAL ADVICE FOR SEXUAL CONNECTION AND HEALING OUR SEXUAL WOUNDS

Bass, Ellen, and Laura Davis. *The Courage to Heal: A Guide for Women Survivors of Child Sexual Abuse.* New York: Harper and Row, 1988.

Britton, Patti. *The Art of Sex Coaching: Expanding Your Practice.* New York: W.W. Norton, 2005.

Castleman, Michael. *Great Sex: A Man's Guide to the Secret Principles of Total-Body Sex.* New York: Rodale Books, 2004.

Foley, Sallie, Sally Kope, and Dennis Sugrue. *Sex Matters for Women: A Complete Guide to Taking Care of Your Sexual Self.* Binghamton, N.Y.: Guilford Press, 2002.

Maltz, Wendy. *The Sexual Healing Journey: A Guide for Survivors of Sexual Abuse.* New York: Harper Collins, 1992.

Northrup, Christiane. *Women's Bodies, Women's Wisdom: Creating Physical and Emotional Health and Healing.* New York: Bantam, 1995.

Paget, Lou. *How to Give Her Absolute Pleasure: Totally Explicit Techniques Every Woman Wants Her Man to Know.* New York: Broadway Books, 2000.

Sprinkle, Annie. *Dr. Sprinkle's Spectacular Sex: Make Over Your Love Life with One of the World's Great Sex Experts.* New York: Tarcher, 2005.

Zoldbrod, Aline. *How Your Childhood Shaped Your Sex Life and What to Do about It.* Oakland, Calif.: New Harbinger Publications, 1998.

Sexuality, Spirituality, and Religion

Beattie-Jung, Patricia, Mary E. Hunt, and Radhika Balakrishnan. *Good Sex: Feminist Perspectives from the World's Religions.* New Brunswick, N.J.: Rutgers University Press, 2001.

Bishop, Clifford. *Sex and Spirit.* Boston: Little, Brown, 1996.

Bonheim, Jalaja. *Aphrodite's Daughters: Women's Sexual Stories and the Journey of the Soul.* New York: Fireside, 1997.

Brock, Rita N. *Journeys by Heart: A Christology of Erotic Power.* New York: Crossroad, 1988.

Eisler, Riane. *Sacred Pleasure: Sex, Myth, and the Politics of the Body.* San Francisco: Harper Collins, 1995.

Gimbutas, Marija. *The Language of the Goddess.* San Francisco: Harper & Row, 1989.

Heyward, Carter. *Touching Our Strength: The Erotic as Power and the Love of God.* New York: Harper Collins, 1989.

Moore, Thomas. *The Soul of Sex: Cultivating Life as an Act of Love.* New York: Harper Collins, 1998.

Savage, Linda E. *Reclaiming Goddess Sexuality: The Power of the Feminine Way.* Carlsbad, Calif.: Hay House, 1999.

Timmerman, Joan H. *Sexuality and Spiritual Growth.* New York: Crossroad, 1992.

Wade, Jenny. *Transcendent Sex: When Lovemaking Opens the Veil.* New York: Paraview Pocket Books, 2004.

Tantra and Other Ways of Understanding Our Sexual Energy

Allione, Tsultrim. *Women of Wisdom*. London: Routledge and Kegan Paul, 1984.

Anand, Margo. *The Art of Sexual Ecstasy: The Path of Sacred Sexuality for Western Lovers*. Los Angeles: Jeremy Tarcher, 1989.

Brennan, Barbara. *Hands of Light: A Guide to Healing Through the Human Energy Field*. New York: Bantam Books, 1987.

Bruyere, Rosalyn. *Wheels of Light: Chakras, Auras and the Healing Energy of the Body*. New York: Fireside, 1994.

Eliade, Mircea. *Shamanism: Archaic Techniques of Ecstasy*. New York: Princeton University Press, 1972.

Emoto, Masaru. *The Hidden Messages in Water*. Hillsboro, Ore.: Beyond Words, 2004.

Hunt, Valerie V. *The Infinite Mind: Science of Human Vibrations of Consciousness*. 3rd ed. Los Angeles: Malibu Publications, 2000.

Ingerman, Sandra. *Medicine for the Earth: How to Transform Personal and Environmental Toxins*. New York: Three Rivers Press, 2000.

Judith, Anodea. *Wheels of Life: A User's Guide to the Chakra System*. Rev. ed. St Paul, Minn.: Llewellan Publications, 2001.

Shaw, Miranda. *Passionate Enlightenment: Women in Tantric Buddhism*. Princeton, N.J.: Princeton University Press, 1994.

Stubbs, Kenneth Ray. *The Essential Tantra: A Modern Guide to Sacred Sexuality*. New York: Jeremy Tarcher, 1999.

What the Experts Say about Women's Sexuality: Research, Surveys, and Smart Critiques

Daniluk, Judith C. *Women's Sexuality Across the Life Span*. Binghamton, N.Y.: Guilford Press, 1998.

Davis, Katherine Bement. *Factors in the Sex Lives of Twenty-two Hundred Women*. New York: Harper & Brothers, 1929.

Ellison, Carol. *Women's Sexualities: Generations of Women Speak about Sexual Self Acceptance.* San Francisco: New Harbinger, 2000.

Eriksen, Julia A. *Kiss and Tell: Surveying Sex in the Twentieth Century.* Cambridge, Mass.: Harvard University Press, 1999.

Irvine, Janice. *Disorders of Desire: Sex and Gender in Modern American Sexology.* Philadelphia: Temple University Press, 1990.

Freud, Sigmund. "Three Contributions to the Theory of Sex." In *The Basic Writings of Sigmund Freud.* Edited and translated by A. A. Brill. New York: Random House, 1938.

Hicks, Karen. "Women's Sexual Problems: A Guide to the New View Approach." www.medscape.com/view/program/3437. 2004.

Hite, Shere. *The Hite Report: A Nationwide Study of Female Sexuality.* New York: Macmillan, 1976.

Jung, Carl G. *The Archetypes and the Collective Unconscious.* Translated by R.F.C. Hall. New York: Pantheon Books, 1959.

Kaplan, Helen Singer. *Disorders of Sexual Desire.* New York: Brunner/ Mazel, 1979.

Kinsey, Alfred C., Wardell B. Pomeroy, and Clyde E. Martin. *Sexual Behavior in the Human Male.* Philadelphia: W. B. Saunders Co., 1948.

Kinsey, Alfred C., Wardell B. Pomeroy, Clyde E. Martin, and Paul H. Gebhard. *Sexual Behavior in the Human Female.* Philadelphia: W.B. Saunders Co., 1953.

Kleinplatz, Peggy J., ed. *New Directions in Sex Therapy: Innovations and Alternatives.* Philadelphia: Brunner-Routledge, 2001.

Laumann, Edward O., John H. Gagnon, Robert T. Michael, and Stuart Michaels. *The Social Organization of Sexuality: Sexual Practices in the United States.* Chicago: University of Chicago Press, 1994.

Laumann, Edward O., Anthony Paik, and Raymond Rosen. "Sexual Dysfunction in the United States: Prevalence and Predictors." *Journal of the American Medical Association* 281 (Feb. 10, 1999): 537–44.

Loe, Meika. *The Rise of Viagra: How the Little Blue Pill Changed Sex in America.* New York: New York University Press, 2004.

Mosher, Clelia Duel. *The Mosher Survey: Sexual Attitudes of 45 Victorian Women.* Edited by James MaHood and Kristine Wenburg. New York: Arno Press, 1980.

Masters, William H., and Virginia E. Johnson. *Human Sexual Response.* Boston: Little, Brown, 1966.

Ogden, Gina. *Sexuality and Spirituality in Women's Relationships: Preliminary Results of an Exploratory Survey.* Wellesley, Mass.: Wellesley College Center for Research on Women, 2002.

Reich, Wilhelm. *The Function of the Orgasm.* Translated by Vincent R. Carfagno. New York: Farrar, Straus and Giroux, 1973.

Tiefer, Leonore, and Ellyn Kaschak, eds. *A New View of Women's Sexual Problems.* Binghamton, N.Y.: Haworth Press, 2001.

Tolman, Deborah L. *Dilemmas of Desire. Teenage Girls Talk about Sexuality.* Cambridge, Mass.: Harvard University Press, 2003.

Whipple, Beverly, John D. Perry, and Alice K. Ladas. *The G Spot: And Other Discoveries about Human Sexuality.* Rev. ed. New York: Owl, 2005.

Whipple, Beverly, Gina Ogden, and Barry Komisaruk. "Physiological Correlates of Imagery-Induced Orgasm in Women." *Archives of Sexual Behavior* 21, no. 2 (1992): 121–133.

Chapter 2 contains research methodology from the author's article, "Sexuality and spirituality in women's relationships: Preliminary results of an exploratory survey." Working Paper 405. Wellesley College Center for Research on Women (2002).

Chapters 5 and 19 contain material from the author's chapter, "Integrating Sexuality and Spirituality: A Group Approach to Women's Sexual Dilemmas," in *New Directions in Sex Therapy: Innovations and Alternatives*, edited by Peggy J. Kleinplatz (Philadelphia: Brunner-Routledge, 2001), pp. 322–346.

Chapter 9 contains material from the author's article, "Sex and Spirit: The Healing Connection," in *New Age* (1999, January–February), pp. 78–81, 128–130.

Chapter 17 is adapted from a chapter in the author's book *Sexual Recovery* (Deerfield Beach, Fla.: Health Communications, 1990).

The exercise "Desiderata" in chapter 18 is adapted from an exercise originally developed for the author's book (with Beverly Whipple) *Safe Encounters: How Women Can Say Yes to Pleasure and No to Unsafe Sex* (New York: McGraw-Hill, 1989).

The epilogue is adapted from an article by the author in the Spring/Summer 2003 issue of *Spirituality and Sexuality*.

The poem "For a Woman Who Fears She Is Too Damaged to Love Again" was first published in *Goddessing Regenerated* 15 (Spring 2002).

The cartoon "Extra Virgin Olive Oil" copyright © 2004 by Andy Singer—www.andysinger.com. Used with permission.

Graphic representation of the ISIS Wheel by Megan Nunery and Michaela Kirby. The chakra chart in chapter 14 is based on information from Barbara Brennan's *Hands of Light* (Bantam, 1988), Rosalyn

Bruyere's *Wheels of Light* (Fireside, 1994), and Anodea Judith's *Wheels of Life* (Llewellyn, 1999).

Details of brain research in chapter 11 is based on information from Barry Komisaruk and Beverly Whipple, "Brain Activity (fMRI and PET) during Sexual Response in Women with and without Complete Spinal Cord Injury," in Janet S. Hyde, ed., *Biological Substrates of Human Sexuality* (Washington, D.C.: American Psychological Association, 2005), pp. 109–145.

About the Author

Dr. Gina Ogden has had a distinguished career as a marriage and family therapist, sex therapist, teacher, researcher, and author. She has written five books including *Women Who Love Sex: An Inquiry into the Expanding Spirit of Women's Erotic Experience*. Her nationwide survey, "Integrating Sexuality and Spirituality" (the ISIS Survey), challenges the performance-oriented norms established by Kinsey and other sex researchers. An associate professor of sexology at the Institute for Advanced Study of Human Sexuality in San Francisco, she developed the ISIS findings as a visiting scholar at Harvard University's Radcliffe Institute and Wellesley Centers for Research on Women. She has been a featured guest on numerous radio and television programs, including *Oprah*. She lives in Cambridge, Massachusetts. For more information, visit www.GinaOgden.com.